An Atlas of
Surgical Approaches
to the Bones and Joints
of the Dog and Cat

DONALD L. PIERMATTEI, D.V.M., Ph.D.

Diplomate, American College of Veterinary Surgeons
Professor of Surgery, Department of Clinical Sciences
College of Veterinary Medicine and Biomedical Sciences
Colorado State University, Ft. Collins, Colorado

Illustrations by
F. Dennis Giddings, A.M.I.

An Atlas of Surgical Approaches to the Bones and Joints of the Dog and Cat

THIRD EDITION

W. B. SAUNDERS COMPANY
Harcourt Brace Jovanovich, Inc.
Philadelphia London Toronto Montreal Sydney Tokyo

W. B. SAUNDERS COMPANY
Harcourt Brace Jovanovich, Inc.

The Curtis Center
Independence Square West
Philadelphia, Pennsylvania 19106

Library of Congress Cataloging-in-Publication Data

Piermattei, Donald L.

An atlas of surgical approaches to the bones and joints of the
dog and cat / Donald L. Piermattei : illustrations by F. Dennis
Giddings. — 3rd ed.

    p.   cm.

Includes bibliographical references and index.

ISBN 0–7216–1012–9

1. Dogs—Surgery—Atlases.   2. Cats—Surgery—Atlases.
   3. Veterinary surgery—Atlases.   4. Veterinary
   orthopedics—Atlases.   I. Title.

SF981.P54   1993

636.7′0897471–dc20   92–25778

An Atlas of Surgical Approaches to the Bones and Joints of the Dog and Cat, 3rd edition
                            ISBN 0–7216–1012–9

Printed in the United States of America.

Last digit is the print number: 9   8   7   6   5   4   3   2   1

Dedicated to those veterinary surgeons
who pioneered the anatomic approach to surgery
and made this volume possible, especially WOB and RBH.

Preface

In the preface to the first edition of this atlas, which appeared 26 years ago, we stated "in the course of several years' experience teaching small animal surgery to veterinary students, a need for well-illustrated material on the surgical anatomy of the skeletal system became very apparent. . . . It is our hope, therefore, that this book will fill a void in the student's and the practitioner's bookshelves and allow them to have available in one place directions for approaches to all bones." Although many things have changed in veterinary orthopedic surgery in the intervening years, the above statements still reflect the reason for, and the goal of, this third edition. We have done everything in our power to improve this version to meet this goal.

The most obvious changes in the current edition are the drawings, each one of which is a new rendering by F. Dennis Giddings. I am sure that every reader will appreciate the clarity, realism, and beautiful detail of the new plates. Additionally, Dennis was invaluable in helping ensure the anatomic accuracy of each drawing and a constant encouragement in the long and arduous revision process.

A larger variety of approaches to the long bones and joints are depicted in highly detailed and labeled drawings, allowing a choice of approaches to fit the clinical situation or personal preference of the surgeon. The largest increase in the number of approaches is in the joints, reflecting the increased importance of reconstructive joint surgery in areas where leash laws have resulted in fewer fractures to roaming dogs. Other changes have been made to make the book easier to use and more complete. The primary indications are listed for each approach, and cross referencing ("Alternative/Combination Approaches") allows easy comparison of approaches to the same area or the combination of approaches to treat multiple injuries. Each approach has one plate number, no matter how many parts, and thus can be referenced by the plate number rather than by page. All the approaches except those for the lower limbs have been drawn using the left limb in order to simplify the use of *Miller's Anatomy of the Dog* (Evans HE, Christensen GC, 2nd ed. Philadelphia, W. B. Saunders Co., 1979). The right side was used for approaches to the lower limbs in deference to the preponderance of lower limb injuries to the racing Greyhound.

Section I has been expanded and revised to reflect current practice. This section suggests and illustrates standard surgical instruments useful for performing open approaches to the bones and joints in small animals. Also covered are recommendations for aseptic technique as it applies to orthopedic procedures, and many suggestions are made for appropriate draping procedures. Ancillary procedures such as osteotomies and tenotomies that are a routine part of many approaches are covered here so that they do not have to be included in the description of each approach. Also included is a brief illustrated review of surgical principles involved in the typical approach and a short section on musculoskeletal anatomy.

Anatomic nomenclature has been revised to reflect current *Nomina Anatomica Veterinaria* terminology and to be consistent with *Miller's Anatomy of the Dog,* cited above. I also want to acknowledge the help of Professor Michael J. Shively, Department of Veterinary Anatomy, Texas A&M University, for his most incisive and helpful critiques in this area. At the same time I must add that in a few cases widely accepted and understood surgical terms have been used where in my judgment they were more useful than official names, and I bear responsibility for these excursions. In keeping with previous editions, anatomically descriptive names have been used for each approach to avoid use of eponyms, and in the face of increasing numbers of approaches to the same area, some of the names used in previous editions have been changed to allow more precise description. Although an attempt was made to cite the original source for each approach, in many cases this was not traceable, and for any omissions or errors I ask your understanding.

Thanks are due to many people for their help and support, primarily to my wife Marcia, and to Linda Mills, Editor, and the entire production staff of W. B. Saunders Company, who were, as always, patient and helpful.

DONALD L. PIERMATTEI, D.V.M., PH.D.
Fort Collins, Colorado

Contents

Section I ■ General Considerations, 1

Attributes of an Acceptable Approach to a Bone or Joint, 2

Factors to Consider When Choosing an Approach, 2

Aseptic Technique, 3

Surgical Principles, 14

Anatomy, 24

Section II ■ The Head, 31

Approach to the Rostral Shaft of the Mandible, 32

Approach to the Caudal Shaft and Ramus of the Mandible, 34

Approach to the Ramus of the Mandible, 36

Approach to the Temporomandibular Joint, 38

Approach to the Dorsolateral Surface of the Skull, 40

Approach to the Caudal Surface of the Skull, 42

Section III ■ The Vertebral Column, 45

Approach to Cervical Vertebrae 1 and 2 Through a Ventral Incision, 46

Approach to Cervical Vertebrae 1 and 2 Through a Dorsal Incision, 50

Approach to Cervical Vertebrae and Intervertebral Disks 2–7
    Through a Ventral Incision, 54

Approach to the Midcervical Vertebrae Through a Dorsal Incision, 60

Approach to the Caudal Cervical and Cranial Thoracic Vertebrae
    Through a Dorsal Incision, 64

Approach to the Thoracolumbar Vertebrae Through a Dorsal Incision, 70

Approach to the Thoracolumbar Intervertebral Disks Through a
    Dorsolateral Incision, 76

Approach to the Thoracolumbar Intervertebral Disks Through a Lateral Incision, 80

Approach to Lumbar Vertebra 7 and the Sacrum Through a Dorsal Incision, 84

Approach to the Caudal Vertebrae Through a Dorsal Incision, 88

Section IV ■ The Scapula and Shoulder Joint, 91

Approach to the Body, Spine, and Acromion Process of the Scapula, 92

Approach to the Craniolateral Region of the Shoulder Joint, 94

Approach to the Craniolateral Region of the Shoulder Joint by Tenotomy of the Infraspinatus Muscle, 98

Approach to the Caudolateral Region of the Shoulder Joint, 102

Approach to the Caudal Region of the Shoulder Joint, 180

Approach to the Craniomedial Region of the Shoulder Joint, 114

Approach to the Cranial Region of the Shoulder Joint, 118

Section V ■ The Thoracic Limb, 122

Approach to the Proximal Shaft of the Humerus, 124

Approach to the Shaft of the Humerus Through a Craniolateral Incision, 128

Approach to the Shaft of the Humerus Through a Medial Incision, 132

Approach to the Distal Shaft of the Humerus Through a Craniolateral Incision, 138

Approach to the Distal Shaft and Supracondylar Region of the Humerus Through a Medial Incision, 142

Approach to the Lateral Aspect of the Humeral Condyle and Epicondyle, 146

Approach to the Lateral Humeroulnar Part of the Elbow Joint, 150

Approach to the Supracondylar Region of the Humerus and the Caudal Humeroulnar Part of the Elbow Joint, 154

Approach to the Humeroulnar Part of the Elbow Joint by Osteotomy of the Tuber Olecrani, 158

Approach to the Elbow Joint by Osteotomy of the Proximal Ulnar Diaphysis, 164

Approach to the Head of the Radius and Lateral Parts of the Elbow Joint, 168

Approach to the Head of the Radius and Humeroradial Part of the Elbow Joint by Osteotomy of the Lateral Humeral Epicondyle, 172

Approach to the Medial Humeral Epicondyle, 176

Approach to the Medial Aspect of the Humeral Condyle and the Medial Coronoid Process of the Ulna by an Intermuscular Incision, 178

Approach to the Medial Aspect of the Humeral Condyle and Medial Coronoid Process of the Ulna by Osteotomy of the Medial Humeral Epicondyle, 182

Approach to the Proximal Shaft and Trochlear Notch of the Ulna, 186

Approach to the Tuber Olecrani, 188

Approach to the Distal Shaft and Styloid Process of the Ulna, 190

Approach to the Head and Proximal Metaphysis of the Radius, 192

Approach to the Shaft of the Radius Through a Medial Incision, 196

Approach to the Shaft of the Radius Through a Lateral Incision, 200

Approach to the Distal Radius and Carpus Through a Dorsal Incision, 204

Approach to the Distal Radius and Carpus Through a Palmaromedial Incision, 206

Approach to the Accessory Carpal Bone and Palmarolateral Carpal Joints, 210

Approaches to the Metacarpal Bones, 214

Approach to the Proximal Sesamoid Bones, 216

Approaches to the Phalanges and Interphalangeal Joints, 218

Section VI ▪ The Pelvis and Hip Joint, 221

Approach to the Wing of the Ilium and Dorsal Aspect of the Sacrum, 222

Approach to the Ilium Through a Lateral Incision, 224

Approach to the Ventral Aspect of the Sacrum, 228

Approach to the Craniodorsal Aspect of the Hip Joint Through a
    Craniolateral Incision, 230

Approach to the Dorsal Aspect of the Hip Joint Through an Intergluteal Incision, 236

Approach to the Craniodorsal and Caudodorsal Aspects of the Hip Joint by Osteotomy
    of the Greater Trochanter, 240

Approach to the Craniodorsal and Caudodorsal Aspects of the Hip Joint by Tenotomy
    of the Gluteal Muscles, 246

Approach to the Caudal Aspect of the Hip Joint and Body of the Ischium, 248

Approach to the Os Coxae, 252

Approach to the Ventral Aspect of the Hip Joint of the Ramus of the Pubis, 254

Approach to the Pubis and Pelvic Symphysis, 258

Approach to the Ischium, 262

Section VII ▪ The Hindlimb, 264

Approach to the Greater Trochanter and Subtrochanteric Region of the Femur, 266

Approach to the Shaft of the Femur, 270

Approach to the Distal Femur and Stifle Joint Through a Lateral Incision, 272

Approach to the Stifle Joint Through a Lateral Incision, 276

Approach to the Stifle Joint Through a Medial Incision, 278

Approach to the Stifle Joint with Bilateral Exposure, 282

Approach to the Distal Femur and Stifle Joint by Osteotomy of the
    Tibial Tuberosity, 286

Approach to the Lateral Collateral Ligament and Caudolateral Part of
    the Stifle Joint, 288

Approach to the Stifle Joint by Osteotomy of the Origin of the
    Lateral Collateral Ligament, 290

Approach to the Medial Collateral Ligament and Caudomedial Part
    of the Stifle Joint, 292

Approach to the Stifle Joint by Osteotomy of the Origin of the
    Medial Collateral Ligament, 296

Approach to the Shaft of the Tibia, 298

Approach to the Lateral Malleolus and Talocrural Joint, 302

Approach to the Medial Malleolus and Talocrural Joint, 304

Approach to the Tarsocrural Joint by Osteotomy of the Medial Malleolus, 306

Approach to the Calcaneus, 308

Approach to the Calcaneus and Plantar Aspects of the Tarsal Bones, 310
Approach to the Lateral Bones of the Tarsus, 312
Approach to the Medial Bones of the Tarsus, 314
Approach to the Proximal Sesamoid Bones, 314
Approaches to the Phalanges and Interphalangeal Joints, 314
Approach to the Metatarsal Bones, 316

References, 319

Index, 321

General Considerations

- ■ Attributes of an Acceptable Approach to a Bone or Joint

- ■ Factors to Consider when Choosing an Approach

- ■ Aseptic Technique

- ■ Surgical Principles

- ■ Anatomy

Attributes of an Acceptable Approach to a Bone or Joint

The bones and joints must be exposed in a manner that ensures the preservation of the anatomic and physiologic functions of the area invaded. Major blood vessels, nerves, ligaments, and tendons must be avoided or protected. Maximal use must be made of muscle separation, with incision of muscles being avoided whenever possible. Transection of muscle bellies must be kept at an absolute minimum; tenotomy or osteotomy of the muscles at their origin or insertion is much preferred. Skin incisions must be made in such a manner that the vascular supply to the incisions is not impaired and so that underlying implants such as bone plates do not create tension on the skin closure. No pedicles or sharp angles should exist in the incision, because these points commonly undergo avascular necrosis and produce excessive scar formation. A cosmetically acceptable scar should be the goal when operating on pet animals.

In general, the procedure should not add unnecessary trauma to that which the injured area has already sustained. Although the incision may be longer, an adequately large exposure is, in the final analysis, less traumatic than a smaller exposure. With the smaller approach, the surgeon tends to exert excessive pressure when retracting muscles, which directly injures the muscle and also impairs circulation to the area.

Factors to Consider When Choosing an Approach

THE AREA TO BE EXPOSED

The problem of choosing the best approach is easily solved in some instances. For example, there is only one logical way to expose the midshaft of the femur (see the Approach to the Shaft of the Femur, Plate 69), and therefore the decision is easily made. Other areas do not lend themselves to such clear-cut answers. In some instances, the choice is purely a matter of the surgeon's personal preference. The area of the hip joint perhaps illustrates this best, there being many choices for exposure of this general area. Ultimately, it rests with the surgeon to try all approaches and to adapt those most suitable.

The exposure required for bone plating is generally more extensive than for bone-pinning techniques. In this instance, it may be useful or necessary to combine two or more of the approaches illustrated. This is discussed further in the section on "The Type of Fracture or Luxation," below.

BREED, SIZE, AND CONFORMATION OF THE ANIMAL

The area of the hip may also be used to illustrate the relationship of the animal's physique to the problem. We are speaking here not only of the size, but also of the body type and the degree of obesity of the patient. Chondrodystrophied breeds are a particular challenge. The shapes and contours of many muscles in the limbs are distorted, and close attention is required to ensure that you end up where you really want to be.

The obese patient is also a serious problem for the surgeon, for it is difficult to identify muscles when their fascial sheaths are obscured by fat. The only help for this problem is to dissect fat off the deep fascia with the skin to allow better visualization of the underlying muscles. A longer skin incision may be required to achieve adequate exposure at the level of the bones.

THE TYPE OF FRACTURE OR LUXATION

Multiple injuries will require multiple approaches or perhaps a combination of methods. By scanning the approaches to various areas of a bone, one can easily note those which lend themselves to combining. An example might be a combination of one of the procedures for the hip or pelvis with the Approach to the Shaft of the Femur (Plate 69). The most likely alternative/combination approaches are listed for each procedure.

ASSOCIATED SOFT-TISSUE DAMAGE OR INFECTION

When a choice of approaches exists, the extent and location of associated injuries can influence the choice of approach. An attempt is always made to avoid exposing bone through an existing skin wound or sinus tract. The purpose of this is to prevent the transfer of infected or infective material to the bone and the surrounding deep structures. The same reasoning is applied to open (compound) fractures of more than a few hours' duration. When there is no alternative to approaching through such an area, the wound must be meticulously debrided and lavaged. It is then prepared again for surgery and redraped, and fresh gloves and instruments are used for the fracture repair.

Aseptic Technique

The keystone upon which success or failure of open bone and joint surgery rests is meticulous devotion to the ritual of *aseptic technique*. True enough, gentle handling of tissues and an anatomically sound approach are of utmost importance, but they go for nought in the presence of wound infection or osteomyelitis. The incidence of these sequelae can be reduced to less than 3% by attention to rigid asepsis and the proper use of antibiotics. In clean cases, where no contamination or infection is suspected, a large dose of a bactericidal antibiotic (e.g., cephalosporin, penicillin) is given intravenously at the time of anesthesia and repeated in 90 minutes. No antibiotics are given postoperatively. If contamination or infection is suspected, or if serious tissue damage is noted during surgery, then antibiotics are continued several days postoperatively. It must be understood that to be effective at the time of surgery, the antibiotic must be given preoperatively with sufficient time to allow effective serum levels of the drug to be present.

A detailed discussion of the methods of sterilization of packs, gowns, and other supplies is beyond the scope of this book. In general, autoclaving at 250°F and 15-lb pressure and with a contact time of 12 to 15 minutes is the most practical way of sterilizing instruments and cloth materials such as drapes and gowns. Sterilizer indicators* that undergo a color change when exposed to proper sterilization conditions should be used in *every pack*. Total time in the autoclave is different from contact time; total time is that which is sufficient for steam penetration of the largest pack for the minimum contact time of 12 to 15 minutes. Sterilizer indicators are the only means of establishing the correct total time. Ethylene oxide is also a very useful sterilization method, because it allows sterilization of items that would be damaged by heat and therefore allows the use of electric drills and other hardware store items in surgery.

Proper skin preparation, positioning, and draping of the patient are critical elements of aseptic technique that are frequently neglected. For all procedures on limbs, including

---

*Steam-Clox, Aseptic-Thermo Indicator Co., North Hollywood, CA.

the hip or shoulder region, a stockinette draping procedure is advised. Draping the whole limb in sterile, double-thickness stockinette allows the limb to be handled by the surgeon and manipulated in any way necessary. When reducing fractures, the need for alignment of the total limb in all planes is obvious. When reducing luxations, the whole limb can be used to supply additional leverage or torque to aid in reduction.

The limb is clipped circumferentially from the groin or axillary area with a #40 blade and electric clippers, to some distance distal to the proposed skin incision. For approaches to the hip or shoulder, the clipping extends proximally to the midline of the back. When the approach is below the elbow or stifle, the clipping usually starts just above the toes and extends proximally only to the elbow or stifle area. Adhesive tape is applied to the toes or foot to form a stirrup from which the leg can be suspended. The remaining unclipped area is covered with gauze or a rubber plastic glove and adhesive tape (Figure 1A and B).

The animal is next placed on the surgery table with the clipped leg uppermost and the leg suspended by adhesive tape attached to the stirrup and to an infusion stand or a hook in the ceiling (Figure 2). A 45- to 60-degree angle is adequate to allow skin disinfection and draping.

Povidone iodine* ("organic iodine") or chlorhexidine† preparations have proven most efficacious for disinfection of the patient's skin. Using sterile gauze sponges immersed in surgical scrub preparation diluted 50% with water, the patient's skin is scrubbed, starting in the area of the incision and working outward to the limits of the clipped area. After 1 minute of scrubbing, the suds are wiped off with dry, sterile sponges. Again, the wiping starts in the area of the incision and proceeds toward the periphery

---

*Betadine surgical scrub and Betadine antiseptic solution, Purdue-Frederick Co., Norwalk, CT.
†Nolvasan surgical scrub, Fort Dodge Laboratories, Fort Dodge, IO; Hibiclens skin cleanser, Stuart Pharmaceuticals, Wilmington, DE.

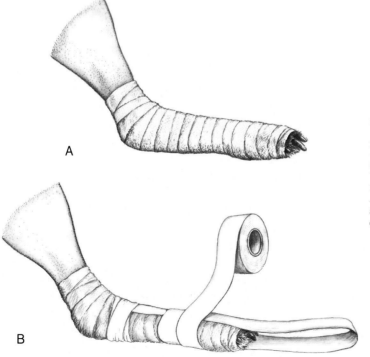

■ Figure 1

A. The unclipped portion of the lower limb is covered with roller gauze bandage or a rubber plastic glove from the toes proximally to the clipped area. **B.** Adhesive tape is used to make a stirrup and to cover the gauze or glove.

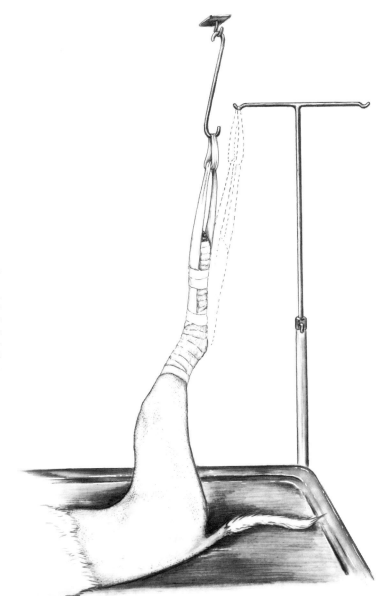

■ **Figure 2**

Suspension of the clipped limb preparatory to skin disinfection. An infusion stand or a hook in the ceiling is used. Adhesive tape can be run directly to the infusion stand from the tape stirrup, but an elongated S-shaped metal rod is interposed between the ceiling and the foot.

of the clipped area. This cycle is repeated five times, and after the final rinse the whole area is sprayed or wiped with 70%–80% isopropyl alcohol, which is allowed to stand and dry on the skin. The same materials are also highly effective for the scrubbing of the surgeon's hands.

The animal is now ready for draping, as soon as the surgeon or assistant is gowned and gloved. Four sterile towels are first placed around the leg at the groin or axillary region (Figure 3). The circulating assistant now grasps the leg on the unprepped area and cuts

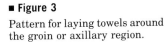

■ **Figure 3**

Pattern for laying towels around the groin or axillary region.

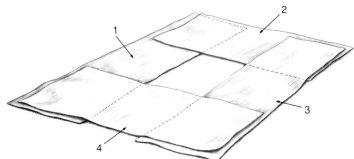

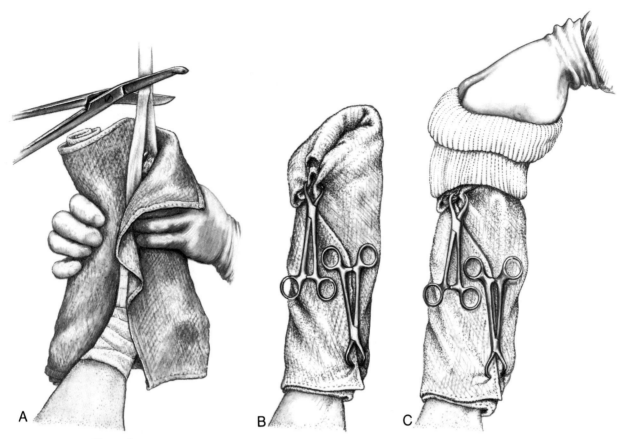

■ **Figure 4**

A. The surgeon grasps the suspended foot through a sterile towel that has been folded and rolled. The suspending tape is cut close to the foot by the technician. **B.** The towel is wrapped around the foot, taking care to cover all of the unprepped area. After folding the towel over the toes, it is secured to the limb with towel clamps. **C.** The surgeon grasps the foot through a sterile, double-thickness, rolled stockinette.

the suspending tape while holding the leg in position. The surgeon grasps the foot through a sterile towel that has been partially rolled (Figure 4A), and then wraps the towel around the unprepped area, while holding the limb up and away from the table. The towel is folded over the toes and secured with towel clamps (Figure 4B). Now the rolled stockinette is placed over the foot (Figure 4C) and unrolled down the leg, taking care not to touch any unprepped areas in the process. When the stockinette meets the towels, the two are joined together and attached to the skin with towel forceps (Figure 5A). A method for the hip or shoulder region is shown in Figure 5B and C. (The stockinette is previously prepared and sterilized. Cut the stockinette twice as long as the leg, using a suitable diameter for the thigh or brachium. Pull half the stockinette inside the other half and tie or tape the cut ends together to make an elongated bag. Roll the uncut end toward the closed end as if rolling a stocking. Wrapping and sterilizing complete the preparation.)

The leg can now be allowed to rest on the table, atop the sterile towels. If the towel under the leg does not cover the table top, a fifth towel is added (Figure 6). The animal and table are next covered with a large fenestrated drape with the stockinette-draped limb protruding through the fenestration. The large drape is accordion-folded to allow

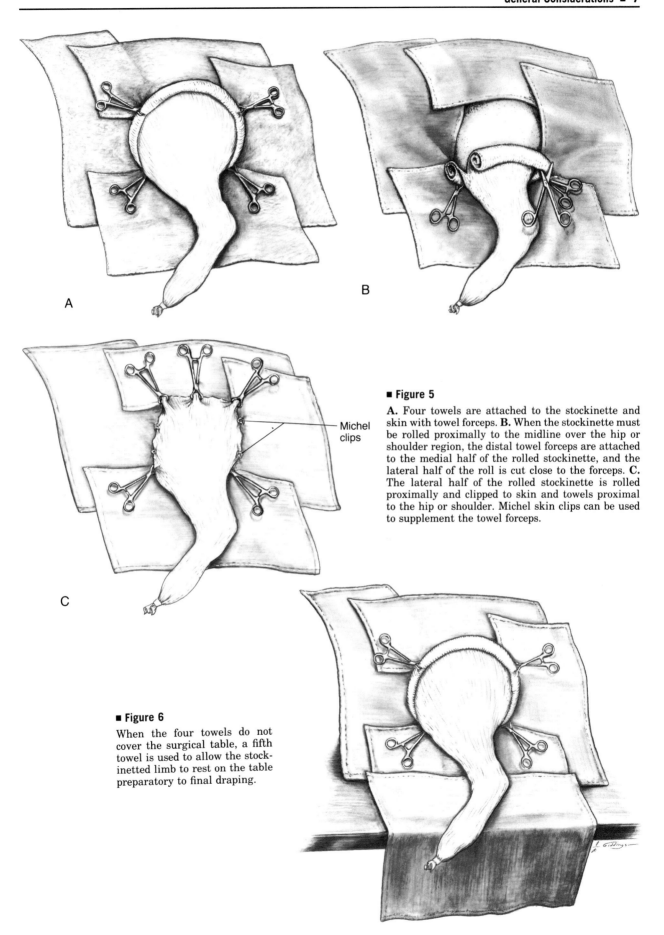

Michel clips

■ **Figure 5**

A. Four towels are attached to the stockinette and skin with towel forceps. **B.** When the stockinette must be rolled proximally to the midline over the hip or shoulder region, the distal towel forceps are attached to the medial half of the rolled stockinette, and the lateral half of the roll is cut close to the forceps. **C.** The lateral half of the rolled stockinette is rolled proximally and clipped to skin and towels proximal to the hip or shoulder. Michel skin clips can be used to supplement the towel forceps.

■ **Figure 6**

When the four towels do not cover the surgical table, a fifth towel is used to allow the stockinetted limb to rest on the table preparatory to final draping.

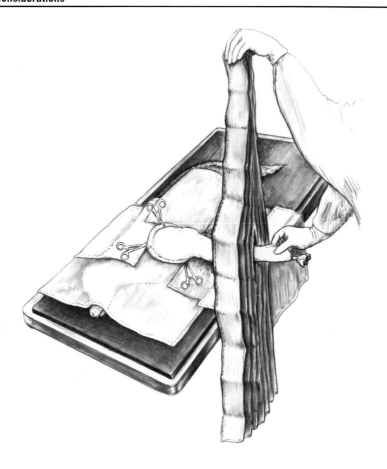

■ **Figure 7**

A fenestrated and fan-folded outer drape is positioned on the stockinetted limb by the surgeon.

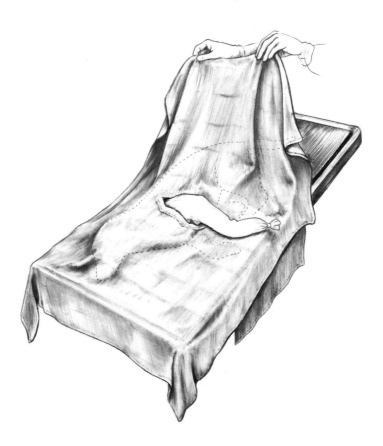

■ **Figure 8**

The left half of the fan-folded drape has been spread and the right half is positioned to complete the draping procedure.

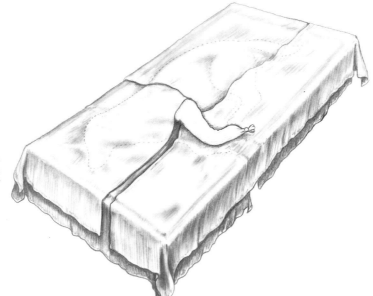

■ **Figure 9**

Four large sheets, used in a manner similar to the initial towels, can be used as an outer drape.

easy opening (Figures 7 and 8). Alternative methods of applying the large drape are available. Four large sheets can be placed around the limb as in Figure 9, or the split-sheet method shown in Figure 10 can be used. The choice of cotton muslin drapes or of impregnated paper materials is one of personal choice. In any case, the large drape should adequately cover the table and the animal. For smaller dogs and cats, this means a drape of 48 × 48 inches (120 × 120 cm) minimum, and for larger breeds, 48 × 72 inches (120 × 180 cm) minimum.

The stockinette is cut over the proposed skin incision. After the skin is incised the cut edges are folded under and are attached to the stockinette with 16-mm Michel skin clips (Figure 11A) or by suturing (Figure 11B). Skin towels can be attached if preferred. Adhesive plastic drapes* have some qualities that make them useful in certain situations, although their cost has somewhat limited their use in veterinary surgery. Because they are both impervious to moisture and transparent, they are useful around areas that are difficult to prepare, such as the feet and the perineal region, and where visualization of a large area is essential during surgery, as in corrective osteotomies. Unfortunately, these drapes do not adhere well to animal skin, even when it is well clipped and scrubbed. Additional adhesive† must be sprayed on the skin to create good adhesion (Figure 12A), but even with this there is considerable loosening of the plastic from the skin if there is much movement of the area during surgery. When used with a stockinette for limb draping, the stockinette is applied as usual, and then a rather large hole is cut in it to expose a generous area of skin for adhesion of the drape. Alternatively, the stockinette is unrolled only part way proximally and the plastic drape is used to cover the rest of the area proximally to the four towels. In the hip and shoulder regions, the stockinette can be attached to the towels medially but not laterally, leaving an open area laterally for the adhesive drape (Figure 12B).

Preparation and draping of the lower limbs present some special problems in aseptic technique. If the surgery is to be in the area of the carpus or tarsus, the limb is clipped

*Barrier Sterile Surgical Incise Drapes, Surgikos Inc., Arlington, TX.
†Vi Drape Adhesive, Deseret Medical Inc., Parke Davis & Co., Sandy, UT.

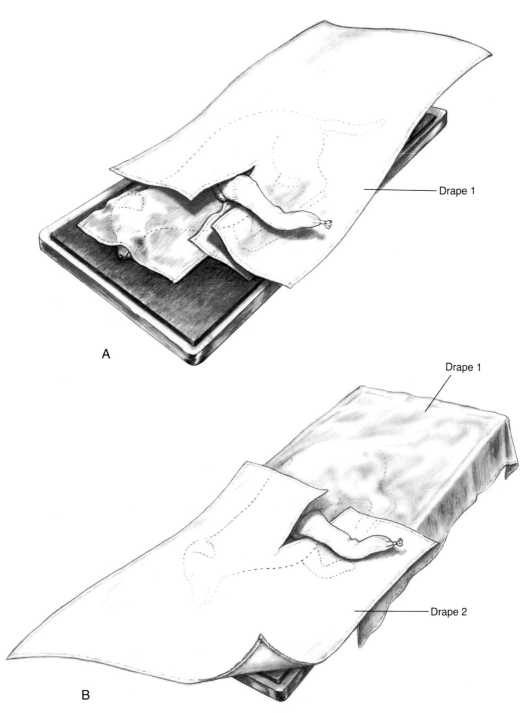

■ **Figure 10**
A. The split-sheet method for an outer drape. Drape 1 is split for a distance of 18 to 24 inches perpendicular to the short end, and the limb is placed on top of one half of the sheet. **B.** Drape 2 is applied in a similar manner so that an 18- to 24-inch overlap of the two sheets occurs.

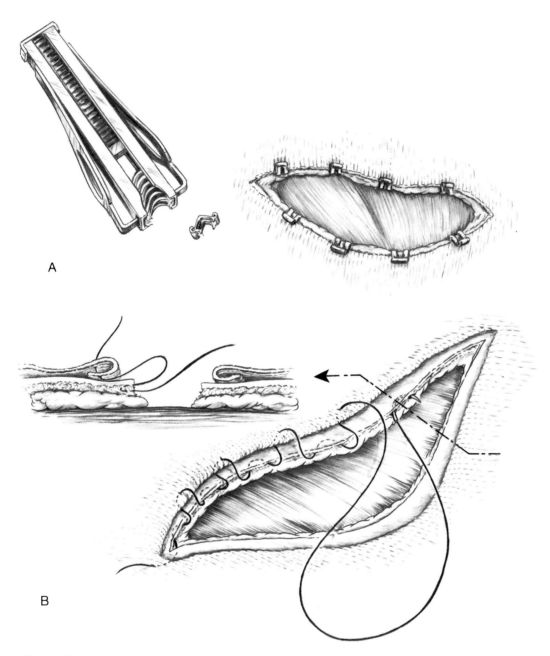

A

B

■ **Figure 11**

A. A skin incision has been made after cutting the stockinette along the proposed line of incision. The stockinette is then clipped to the skin with 16-mm Michel wound clips. **B.** The stockinette can be sutured in place. Note that the suture is placed in the dermis, not the skin, and then through the rolled edge of the stockinette. A taper-point needle is preferred.

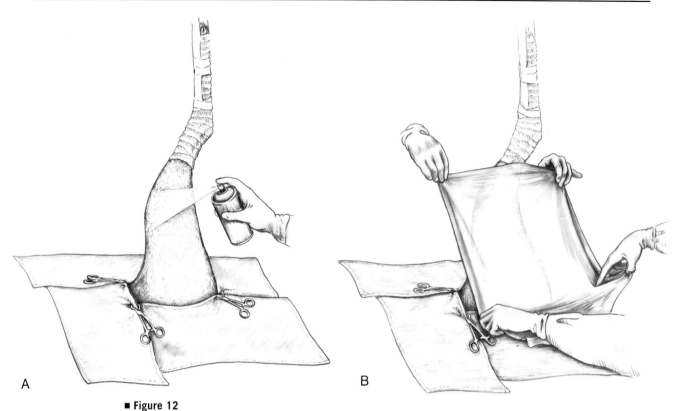

■ **Figure 12**

Placing a transparent plastic adhesive drape. **A.** Sterile adhesive material is sprayed over the prepped area in the region where the adhesive drape will be applied. **B.** After removing the paper backing, the adhesive plastic drape is placed on the prepared skin and pressed in place to stick it to the skin. Stockinette will be placed over the limb distal to the plastic drape.

distally to the proximal phalanges, and the toes are wrapped in adhesive tape to allow suspension of the limb for scrubbing. Because the toes are not prepped, they must be covered intraoperatively in such a way as to prevent strike through of fluids and contamination of the surgical field. As the technician cuts the suspending tape, the surgeon supports the limb by grasping the foot through a sterile towel (Figure 13A) and then placing a stockinette on the limb as described above (Figure 13B). A sterile surgical glove is then used to cover the toes and part of the metacarpus (metatarsus) (Figure 13C). The glove is secured to the foot with a wrapping of sterile elastic bandage material.

If the surgical field extends into the midportion of the metacarpus (metatarsus), the entire foot must be prepared, because there is no way to isolate the field from the rest of the foot. Following clipping, the limb is suspended by a Backhaus towel forceps clamped through a toenail (Figure 14). During scrubbing, particular attention should be paid to the pads, because they are very difficult to cleanse adequately. A final prep of the pads with tincture of iodine is quite effective. The limb and foot are then covered with stockinette as before, but there is now no need for the surgical glove, because the entire foot is prepped. Adhesive plastic drapes can be substituted for stockinette quite effectively, especially when the entire foot is not prepped, because they eliminate the need for placing the surgical glove to prevent strike through.

For incisions on the trunk, neck, and head, the draping technique is considerably simplified. After skin preparation, the area of the incision is delineated by laying four

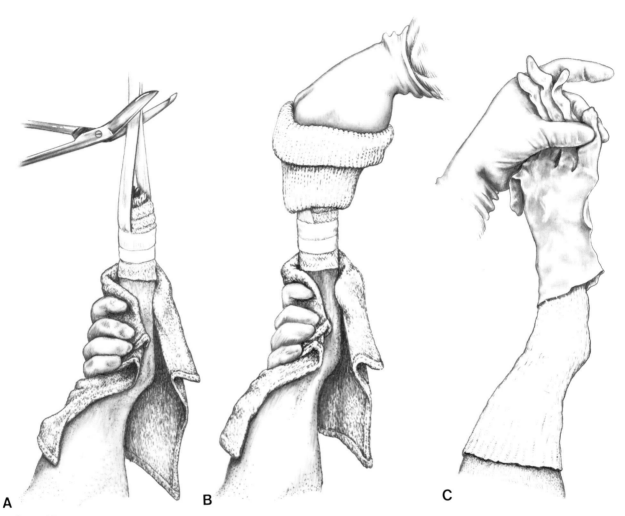

A   B   C

■ Figure 13

Draping the foot when the region of the toes has not been prepped. **A.** The surgeon grasps the suspended foot through a sterile towel. The suspending tape is cut close to the foot by the technician. **B.** The stockinette is unrolled proximally while the limb is supported by the opposite hand. **C.** A sterile glove is placed on the foot so as to cover the unprepped portion and is secured in place with sterile elastic bandage material (Vetrap, Animal Care Products, 3-M, St. Paul, MN). Bandage material, glove, and stockinette are incised over the area of the skin incision.

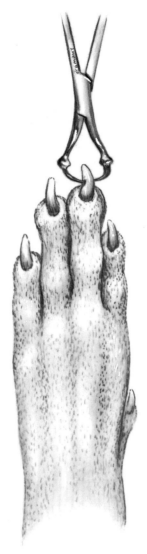

■ Figure 14
When the entire foot is to be prepped, the foot is suspended with a Backhaus towel forceps placed into a toenail.

sterile towels around the area, which are then attached to the skin with towel forceps. The large drape, similar in size to that described above, is simply placed over the area and opened. Skin towels are clipped or sewn to the skin after the skin incision is completed. When using disposable paper drapes, it is often convenient to clip the drape directly to the incised skin and thus dispense with skin towels.

It is a point worth stressing that adequate draping simplifies the workload of the surgeon by eliminating the need to worry about where a hand or instrument may come to rest in an unguarded moment. If the drape is large enough, any area within a reasonable distance from the incision is "safe." The longer the procedure, the more important draping and all other aspects of asepsis become. Procedures lasting longer than 1 hour are significantly more prone to wound infections than are shorter operations.

Surgical Principles

Assuming that aseptic technique is scrupulously practiced, the success or failure of an open approach rests on the surgeon's skill in handling tissues *atraumatically*. Although many of the methods herein described are well known to the experienced surgeon, it is hoped that this review will be useful to the practicing surgeon, in addition to serving as an introduction to this subject for the student.

INCISING AND RETRACTING SKIN AND SUBCUTANEOUS TISSUES

The skin and dermal fascia are incised cleanly and completely before an attempt is made to pick up bleeding vessels. The incision will gape widely when the fascia is completely cut, and subsequent eversion of the cut edges facilitates the clamping of bleeders. Meticulous hemostasis is necessary for optimal skin healing. The use of an electrosurgical apparatus for coagulating smaller bleeders is invaluable as a time saver and as a way of achieving a dry surgical field. Regrettably, this technique is not often enough used by veterinary surgeons.

In most cases, subcutaneous fat is incised on the same line as the skin. The fat is incised down to the deep fascial layer, which lies directly on the muscles. It is usually necessary to bluntly separate fat from fascia by the undermining technique shown in Figure 15. This method allows the skin to be widely retracted with minimal interference with its

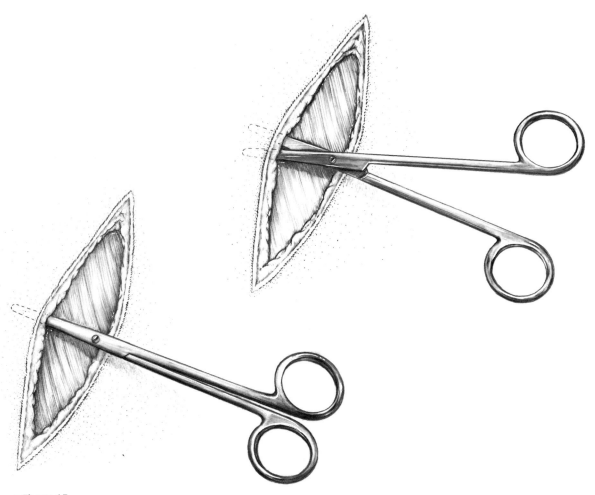

■ **Figure 15**
Undermining skin and subcutaneous fascia and fat by using Mayo scissors and blunt dissection technique.

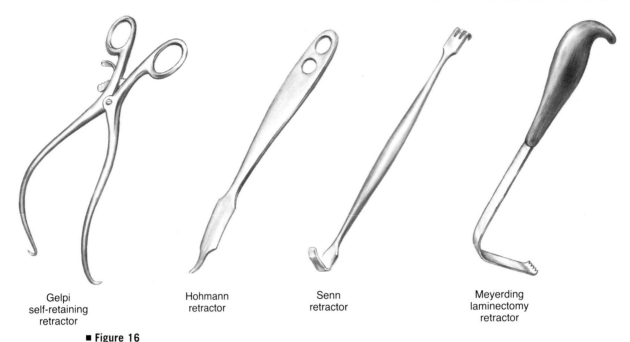

Gelpi
self-retaining
retractor

Hohmann
retractor

Senn
retractor

Meyerding
laminectomy
retractor

■ **Figure 16**

These retractors are representative of types useful in small animal orthopedic surgery.

blood supply and exposes the fascia to allow the visualization necessary for the proposed fascial incision.

Hemostatic (crushing) clamps should never be applied to the cut edges of the skin, and even Allis forceps are best fastened to subcutaneous fascia to avoid possible trauma. The use of retractors is highly encouraged as a means of avoiding tissue damage. Useful examples of these are shown in Figure 16. The Gelpi self-retaining retractor is virtually a third hand for the surgeon working alone. Hohmann and Meyerding laminectomy retractors are particularly valuable in the region of the pelvis and hip joint. When selecting rake-type retractors like the Volkman, Senn, or Mathieu, those with sharp teeth are to be preferred over those with rounded teeth. The points on the latter tend to slip more, resulting in more trauma than the sharp points produce.

Deep fascia may be loosely adherent to the musculature and may actually slide freely over the muscles, as with the fascia lata, or it may be tightly adherent to the deep structures and difficult to separate from the muscle sheaths. The latter condition is particularly true distal to the elbow and the stifle joint.

A method of incising movable fascia to avoid damaging deep structures is depicted in Figure 17. Tightly adherent fascia is incised with the scalpel, with care being taken to make the incisions directly over muscle separations whenever possible. Fascia is rarely retracted by itself, but is usually retracted with the muscles exposed by the fascial incision.

MUSCLE SEPARATION, ELEVATION, AND RETRACTION

Muscles are separated and elevated from the bone in order to obtain exposure of the bone. The incision of muscles is avoided wherever possible, and tenotomy is held to a

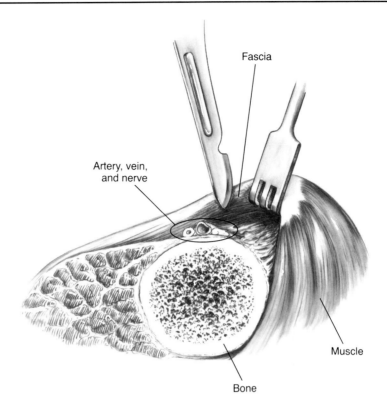

■ Figure 17

Method of incising deep fascia. The muscle sheath is grasped with forceps and lifted to elevate the fascia from deeper structures.

Fascia

Artery, vein, and nerve

Muscle

Bone

minimum. Nothing contributes more to an early return of function than the intelligent and gentle handling of muscles.

Muscles are held against the bone by the deep fascia that surrounds the trunk and limbs like a tube. When this fascia is incised, muscles are relatively free except at their origins and insertions. The space between muscles, called the intermuscular septum, is occupied by rather loose fascial tissue. Bellies of adjacent muscles rarely adhere to one another. Therefore, to separate muscles after the incision of the deep fascia, it is necessary to divide only the intermuscular septa. This is accomplished as shown in Figure 18.

Once the muscles have been separated from one another, they must be elevated and retracted. In some cases, muscles are easily elevated from underlying bone because there are no extensive periosteal attachments in the area. As an example, the bellies of the vastus lateralis and vastus intermedius muscles are easily separated from the shaft of the femur (see Approach to the Shaft of the Femur, Plate 69) by bluntly separating the loose periosteal attachments of the muscular fascia in a manner similar to that shown in Figure 18.

In areas where the muscle is more firmly adherent to the bone, it must be elevated in a different manner. Subperiosteal elevation allows muscle to be freed from bone at its origin or insertion without disturbing the muscle fibers. The periosteum is incised and undermined with a periosteal elevator (Figure 19). A narrow, slightly curved, and sharp elevator such as the Langenbeck or A.S.I.F. pattern works well. Because the periosteum of the dog is rather thin and firmly attached in the area of muscular attachments, its elevation is difficult in skeletally mature animals. In immature animals, the periosteum is tough and thick enough to allow incision and elevation of the intact periosteum.

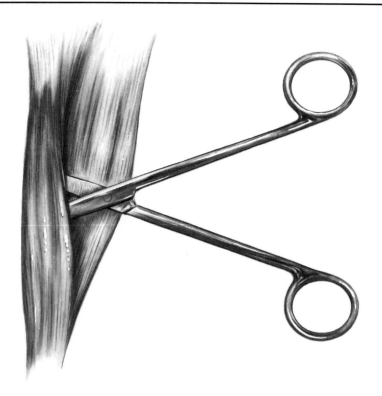

■ **Figure 18**

Blunt dissection of an intermuscular septum.

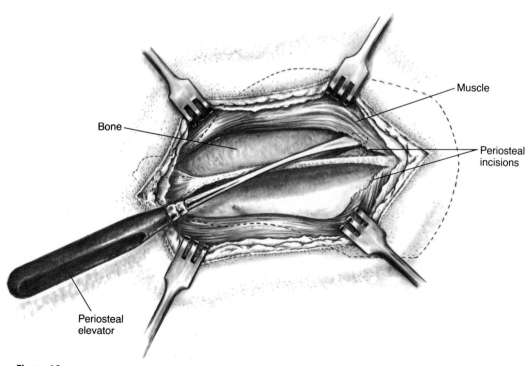

■ **Figure 19**

Subperiosteal elevation of a muscle.

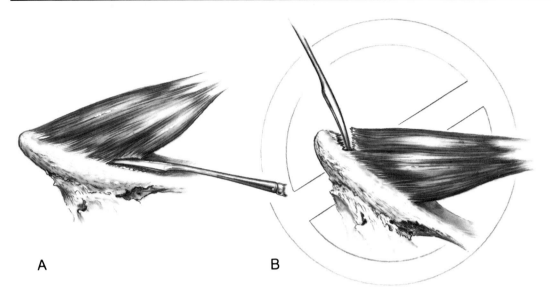

A   B

■ **Figure 20**

Elevation of muscle from bone in a mature animal. **A.** When the elevating instrument and the muscle fibers form a "V" relative to each other, the muscle peels cleanly from the periosteum. **B.** When the elevating instrument and muscle fibers form an "X" relative to each other, the muscle fibers are cut irregularly before they peel away from the bone.

One form of muscular attachment to bone of interest is the fleshy attachment, in which muscular fascia is attached to the periosteum over a large area, as is well illustrated by the origin of the middle gluteal muscle on the iliac wing and crest. Fleshy attachments are elevated by the incision of the fascial connection with the periosteum. The periosteal elevator, scalpel blade, or bone chisel is held almost flat against the bone and the muscle is separated with a "shaving" action. It is important that this elevation be done in the correct direction relative to the direction of the muscle fibers. The elevation should proceed in the same direction as the fibers, because this allows muscle fibers to be peeled off the periosteum of the mature dog with less fraying and tearing than does elevation in the opposite direction (Figure 20). Such areas cannot be sutured back to the bone, but will reattach by fibrosis if the primary tendinous origin or insertion is left intact or sutured.

In some cases, muscles are freed by incising their tendon or aponeurosis of origin or insertion on the bone. This technique is called tenotomy. In some cases, sufficient stump is left attached to the bone so that sutures can be placed to reunite the tendon (see Part E of Plate 23, and Figure 21). Because in some cases the tendons may be too short for convenient suturing, they are sometimes cut close to the bone and reattached directly to the bone with sutures (Figure 22). In other cases, the tendon or aponeurosis is severed close to the bone and no attempt is made at suturing. The best example of this is the elevation of the lumbar muscles from the lumbar vertebrae in the Approach to the Thoracolumbar Vertebrae Through a Dorsal Incision (Plate 17). Finally, the bony insertion of the tendon can be osteotomized to allow reflection of the tendon and muscle (see Plate 74). Osteotomies can be performed with power oscillating or reciprocating saws, hand saws, Gigli wire saws, or osteotomes. Although these bone fragments might be reattached in many ways, some of the most useful are shown in Figures 23 and 24.

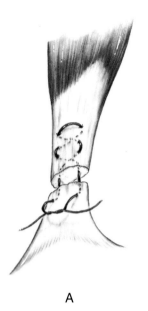

A

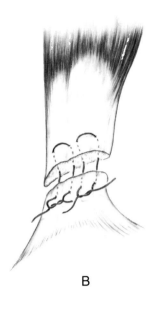

B

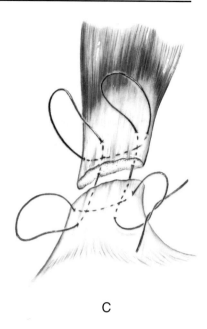

C

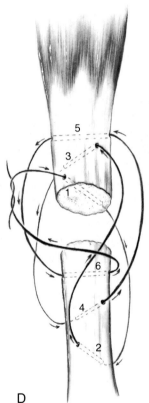

D

■ **Figure 21**

Tendon and ligament suture patterns. **A.** Modified Bunnell-Mayer suture pattern used in a small tendon cut close to the bone. **B.** Horizontal mattress suture pattern used in a large, flat tendon. **C.** The locking-loop (Kessler) suture creates a very secure closure of either tendon or ligament. **D.** The pulley suture is easy to place in small tendons (or ligaments) and has very good holding power. The initial needle passes 1 and 2 are placed in a near–far pattern. Passes 3 and 4 are rotated 120 degrees from 1 and 2 and are placed midway between the near and far positions. Passes 5 and 6 are rotated 120 degrees from 3 and 4 and are placed in the far–near pattern. (After Berg RJ, and Egger EL: *In vitro* comparison of the three loop pulley and locking loop suture patterns for repair of canine weightbearing tendons and collateral ligaments. Vet Surg 15:107–110, 1986.)

■ **Figure 22**

A large tendon cut at its insertion is reattached with a locking-loop suture passed through holes drilled in the bone.

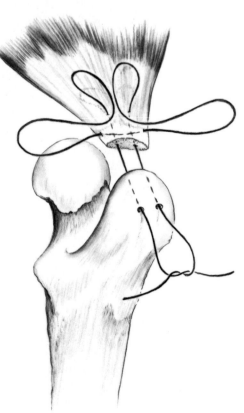

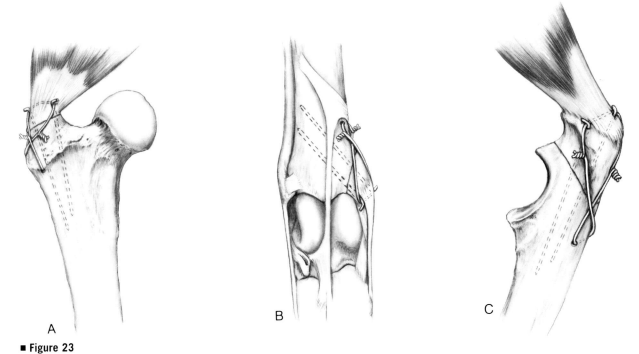

■ **Figure 23**

Examples of two pins or Kirschner wires and tension band wire used to reattach osteotomized bone that is subject to tension forces. **A.** Greater trochanter. **B.** Medial malleolus. **C.** Olecranon.

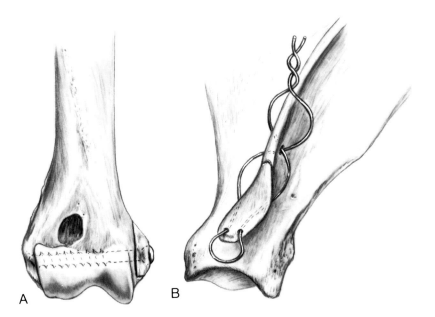

■ **Figure 24**

Other methods of securing osteotomized bone. **A.** A lag screw placed through the medial humeral condyle. No screw threads cross the osteotomy line. **B.** Wire fixation of an osteotomized acromion process on the scapular spine.

After the muscles have been elevated, they are retracted and held with muscle retractors. The retractors shown in Figure 16 are quite adequate, although there are many other types available. At least one self-retaining and one hand-held retractor are necessary for adequate exposure. A person operating without an assistant could well use two self-retaining retractors.

In the course of separating and elevating muscles, many large blood vessels and major nerve trunks will be encountered in the fascial planes between muscles. These structures must obviously be preserved at all cost. The anatomy of the area should be kept firmly in mind or reviewed if necessary before each procedure. See the section, "Anatomy," below for more discussion on this subject.

Whenever possible, the nerve or vessel is retracted with an adjoining muscle; this technique takes advantage of the muscle as padding and also prevents undue stretching of the nerve or vessel. On occasion, these structures must be retracted by themselves in order to achieve adequate exposure of underlying structures. In such a case, the vessel or nerve is carefully freed from its enveloping fascia by blunt dissection. A mosquito hemostat is very useful for this dissection, because its use avoids the accidental severing of structures that is possible with dissection scissors. When the vessel or nerve has been sufficiently loosened, ¼-inch Penrose tubing is passed around the structure and is then used to maintain traction. This practice is considerably less traumatic than retraction with a metal instrument.

CLOSURE

Suture materials have been dramatically improved in their handling qualities and performance in recent years. Catgut has been virtually replaced by synthetic absorbable materials, and the monofilaments have emerged as the nonabsorbable materials of choice. Selection of suture materials and patterns seems to be a highly personal matter with surgeons, and one would have a difficult time arriving at a consensus, but the following selections have served the author well.

Suture Material. *Nonabsorbable.* Any material that is to be buried must be sterilized by steam or ethylene oxide. Chemical sterilization or dispensing from cassettes is not reliable. Monofilament materials such as nylon and polypropylene have a lower infection rate and less local reaction associated with them than do braided materials, and are the choice for most applications where long-lasting strength is important and for skin closure.

Absorbable. Two styles of synthetic materials are available. The first are the braided materials characterized by polyglactin (Vicryl—Ethicon) and polyglycolic acid (Dexon—Davis & Geck). They have pleasant handling qualities and a half-life of about 14 days in situ, and they elicit less local reaction than does catgut. The second synthetic material is polydioxanone (PDS—Ethicon), which is a monofilament material with an in situ half-life of about 50 days. Although its handling qualities are not as good as those of the braided materials, it is a very versatile suture that will maintain its strength long enough for healing in almost any situation. It can therefore replace nonabsorbable material in many cases and thereby decrease the infection rate associated with nonabsorbable materials, especially in the larger sizes.

Joint Capsule. This tissue supports sutures well. Interrupted stitches are generally used because of their reliability and safety. Suture material selection for joint capsule closure is the subject of a wide variety of opinions. Some general rules are:

- When the closure can be made without tension and the capsule is not important in stabilizing the joint, use continuous sutures of small gauge (2-0 to 4-0) absorbable material or an interrupted pattern with nonabsorbable materials.
- If the capsule must be closed under tension or is being imbricated to add stability, use interrupted sutures of nonabsorbable material in sizes 3-0 to 1. The choice of material is not critical; however, monofilament materials such as nylon or polypropylene are not as prone to becoming infected as are the braided materials. It is important with any nonabsorbable material that the suture not penetrate the synovial membrane in an area that would allow the suture to rub on articular cartilage. Such contact will cause erosion of the cartilage. Lembert and mattress patterns allow slight imbrication, whereas the simple interrupted pattern allows edge-to-edge apposition.

Muscles. Sutures tend to cut and pull through this relatively soft tissue. A horizontal mattress pattern offers the best resistance against being pulled out should it be necessary to suture fleshy portions of muscles. The external fascial sheath of the muscle is the strongest part of muscle tissue and thus is most important in supporting sutures.

Tendons and Ligaments. Although tendons are dense and strong because of the longitudinal and parallel arrangement of their fibers, most stitches tend to cut through them. A selection of the most-used patterns is shown in Figure 21. Monofilament material works best in these tissues, because it glides through tissue easily and allows all slack to be removed from the pattern before tying.

Osteotomized bone with tendon or ligaments attached must be securely fixed in place for rapid fracture healing to occur. Because of muscle pull, there is a tendency for these bone fragments to be unstable and for delayed union to occur, with a resulting delay in the limb's return to function. The tension band wire technique illustrated in Figure 23 is a very effective way of overcoming these muscular forces. Lag screw fixation or simple wire sutures can also be used in certain situations, as illustrated in Figure 24.

Deep Fascia. No special precautions need to be taken here, because this tissue holds sutures well. Simple interrupted or simple running patterns work equally well. The use of synthetic absorbable material combined with good knot-tying technique makes continuous patterns completely practical here.

Subcutaneous Fascia and Dermal Fat. Proper closure of this layer is important for two reasons: (1) the space created by incising and undermining the fat fills with serum unless the space is obliterated, and (2) closure of the fascia can relieve most of the tension on skin sutures. Simple interrupted or continuous patterns are used. The method of placing the suture is illustrated in Figure 25.

Skin. Simple interrupted sutures are the usual choice in the closure of skin, although many prefer one of the mattress patterns—either horizontal or vertical. Interrupted stitches are preferred by most, although continuous intradermal closures using synthetic absorbable sutures have worked well in the hands of the author.

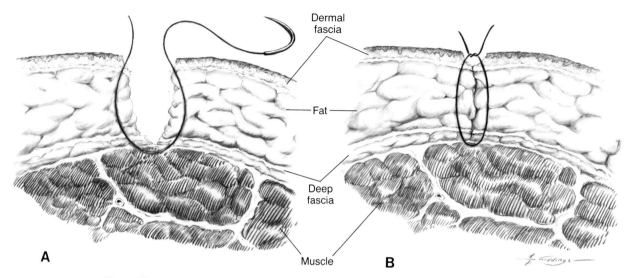

■ Figure 25

Method of placing sutures in subcutis. **A.** Simple stitch engages dermal fascia, fat, and muscular or deep fascia. **B.** When stitch is pulled tight, it apposes all subcutaneous tissues, eliminates dead space, and thereby prevents the formation of serum pockets.

Anatomy

Plates 1 through 5 are included here to provide ready reference to the major muscles, vessels, and nerves of the fore- and hindlimbs. These plates are *not* intended to substitute for detailed study in a suitable anatomy text. For this, these books are highly recommended, although many others are suitable:

Evans HE, Christensen GC: *Miller's Anatomy of the Dog,* 2nd ed. Philadelphia: W. B. Saunders Co., 1979.
Crouch JE: *Text-Atlas of Cat Anatomy.* Philadelphia: Lea & Febiger, 1969.

An experienced surgeon who uses open approaches on a daily basis soon has the anatomy of each one well in mind, but the surgeon who is exposed only occasionally to a given area often will find difficulty in performing in it. A major problem for all, but more so for the less experienced, is the distortion of normal anatomy due to trauma. Subcutaneous tissues and muscles become hemorrhagic and swollen, making identification difficult. In addition, points of origin and insertion of muscles and tendons are often displaced because of fractures. A good grasp of regional anatomy is absolutely essential in these situations.

Do not be apologetic about reviewing the anatomy of a region before surgery. Consider it not an admission of ignorance, but instead the badge of a dedicated and conscientious surgeon who has the welfare of the patient uppermost in mind.

Plate 1

Subcutaneous Musculature of the Canine Forequarter

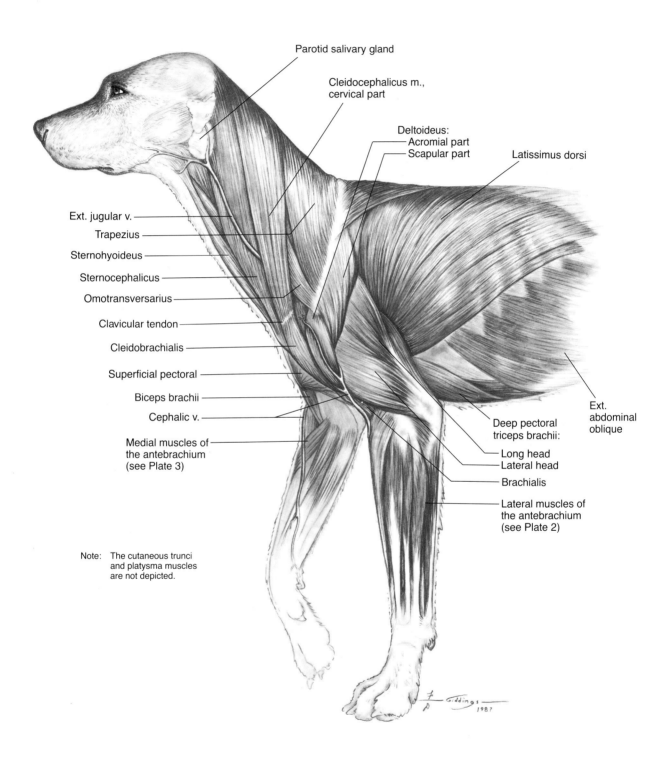

Parotid salivary gland

Cleidocephalicus m., cervical part

Deltoideus:
- Acromial part
- Scapular part

Latissimus dorsi

Ext. jugular v.

Trapezius

Sternohyoideus

Sternocephalicus

Omotransversarius

Clavicular tendon

Cleidobrachialis

Superficial pectoral

Biceps brachii

Cephalic v.

Medial muscles of the antebrachium (see Plate 3)

Ext. abdominal oblique

Deep pectoral triceps brachii:
- Long head
- Lateral head

Brachialis

Lateral muscles of the antebrachium (see Plate 2)

Note: The cutaneous trunci and platysma muscles are not depicted.

25

Plate 2

Deep Musculature of the Canine Thoracic Limb, Lateral View

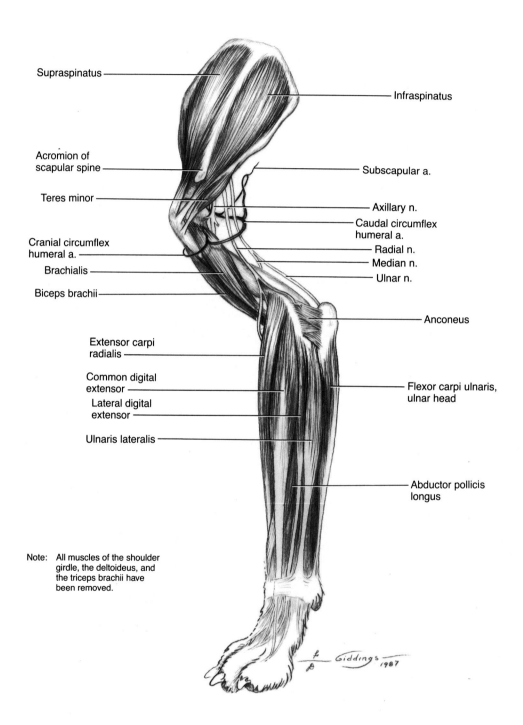

Supraspinatus

Infraspinatus

Acromion of scapular spine

Subscapular a.

Teres minor

Axillary n.

Caudal circumflex humeral a.

Cranial circumflex humeral a.

Radial n.

Brachialis

Median n.

Biceps brachii

Ulnar n.

Anconeus

Extensor carpi radialis

Common digital extensor

Flexor carpi ulnaris, ulnar head

Lateral digital extensor

Ulnaris lateralis

Abductor pollicis longus

Note: All muscles of the shoulder girdle, the deltoideus, and the triceps brachii have been removed.

Giddings 1987

Plate 3

Deep Musculature of the Canine Thoracic Limb, Medial View

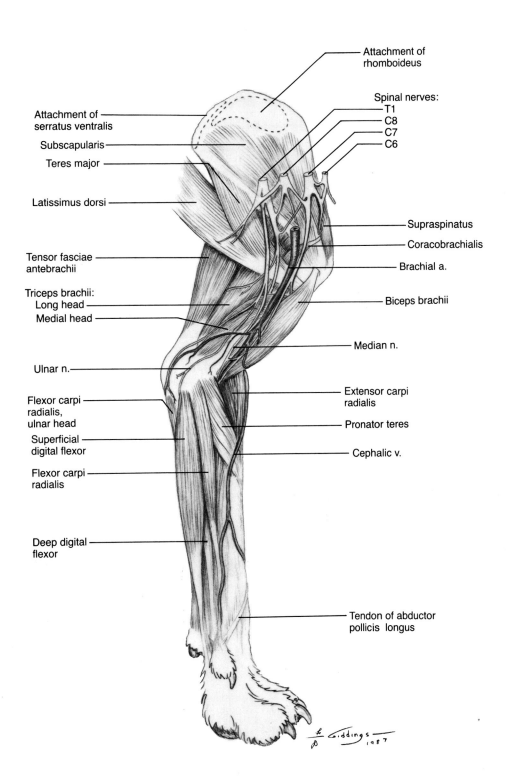

Attachment of rhomboideus

Attachment of serratus ventralis

Subscapularis

Teres major

Latissimus dorsi

Tensor fasciae antebrachii

Triceps brachii:
Long head
Medial head

Ulnar n.

Flexor carpi radialis, ulnar head

Superficial digital flexor

Flexor carpi radialis

Deep digital flexor

Spinal nerves:
T1
C8
C7
C6

Supraspinatus

Coracobrachialis

Brachial a.

Biceps brachii

Median n.

Extensor carpi radialis

Pronator teres

Cephalic v.

Tendon of abductor pollicis longus

Plate 4

Subcutaneous Musculature of the Canine Hindquarter

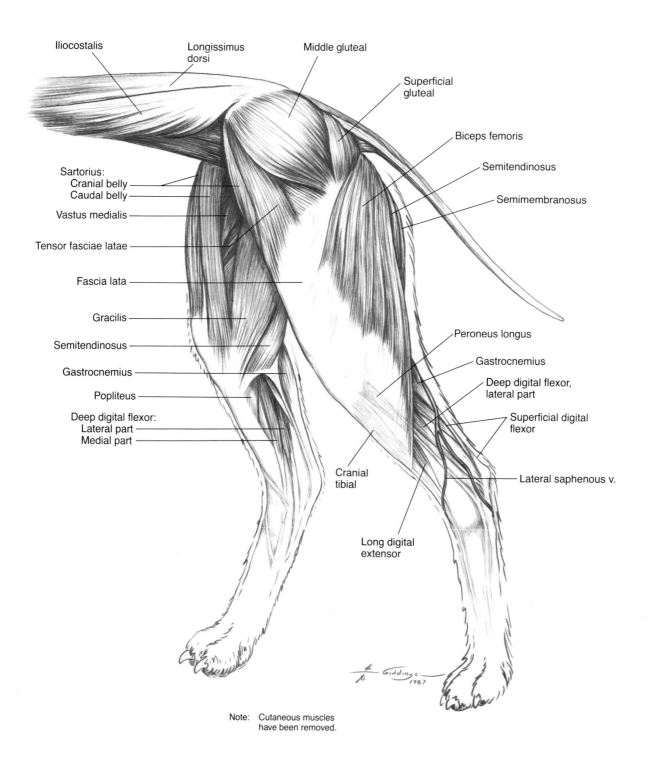

Iliocostalis

Longissimus dorsi

Middle gluteal

Superficial gluteal

Biceps femoris

Semitendinosus

Semimembranosus

Sartorius:
Cranial belly
Caudal belly

Vastus medialis

Tensor fasciae latae

Fascia lata

Gracilis

Semitendinosus

Gastrocnemius

Popliteus

Deep digital flexor:
Lateral part
Medial part

Peroneus longus

Gastrocnemius

Deep digital flexor, lateral part

Superficial digital flexor

Cranial tibial

Lateral saphenous v.

Long digital extensor

Note: Cutaneous muscles have been removed.

Plate 5

Deep Musculature of the Canine Hindquarter

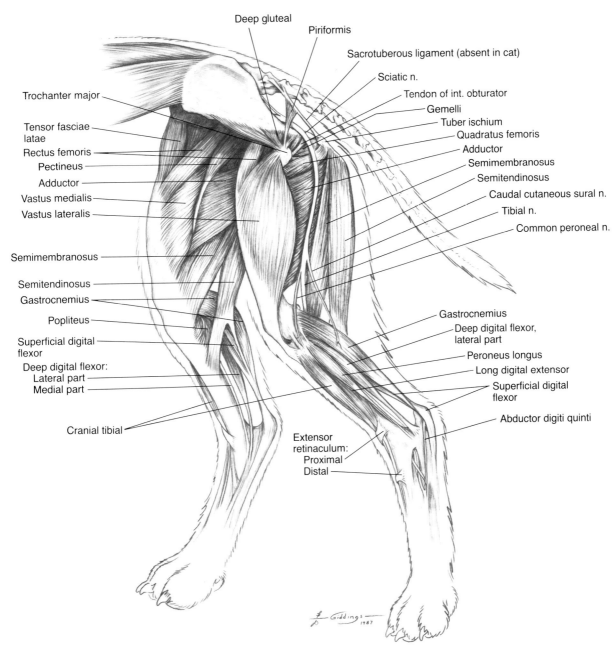

Deep gluteal

Piriformis

Sacrotuberous ligament (absent in cat)

Sciatic n.

Tendon of int. obturator

Gemelli

Tuber ischium

Quadratus femoris

Adductor

Semimembranosus

Semitendinosus

Caudal cutaneous sural n.

Tibial n.

Common peroneal n.

Trochanter major

Tensor fasciae latae

Rectus femoris

Pectineus

Adductor

Vastus medialis

Vastus lateralis

Semimembranosus

Semitendinosus

Gastrocnemius

Popliteus

Superficial digital flexor

Deep digital flexor:
Lateral part
Medial part

Cranial tibial

Gastrocnemius

Deep digital flexor, lateral part

Peroneus longus

Long digital extensor

Superficial digital flexor

Abductor digiti quinti

Extensor retinaculum:
Proximal
Distal

Note: Muscles removed on the lateral side include the middle and deep gluteals, tensor fasciae latae, and biceps femoris. Muscles removed from the medial side include the sartorius and gracilis.

29

The Head

- Approach to the Rostral Shaft of the Mandible

- Approach to the Caudal Shaft and Ramus of the Mandible

- Approach to the Ramus of the Mandible

- Approach to the Temporomandibular Joint

- Approach to the Dorsolateral Surface of the Skull

- Approach to the Caudal Surface of the Skull

Approach to the Rostral Shaft of the Mandible

Based on a Procedure of Rudy [32]

INDICATION

Open reduction of comminuted fractures of the mandible.

ALTERNATIVE/COMBINATION APPROACH

Plate 7

DESCRIPTION OF THE PROCEDURE

A. The skin incision is made slightly lateral to the ventral midline of the mandible from the level of the canine tooth to the level of the molar teeth.

   The flat and very thin platysma muscle will be incised with the subcutaneous fascia, and is then retracted with the fascia and skin.

B. Dorsal retraction of the platysma and skin exposes the shaft of the mandible.

   Subperiosteal elevation of the mylohyoideus muscle can be used to increase the exposure of the medial side of the bone.

CLOSURE

Elevated muscles are sutured to fascia on the surface of the mandible. The platysma and subcutaneous fascia are closed in one layer.

Plate 6
Approach to the Rostral Shaft of the Mandible

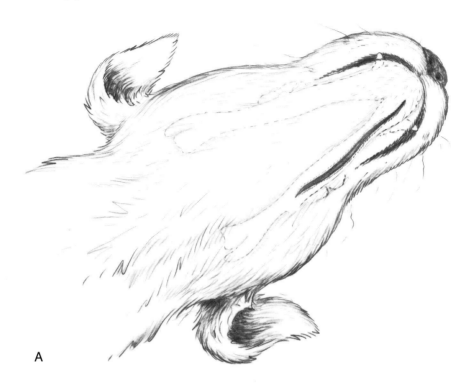

A

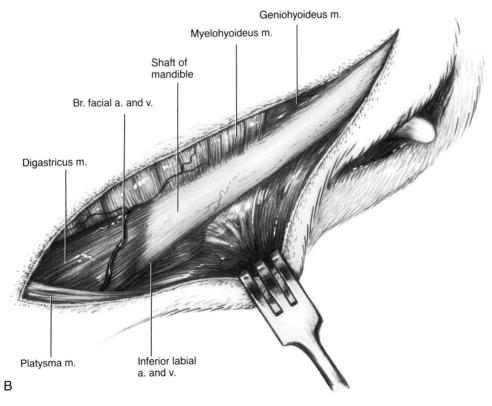

Geniohyoideus m.

Myelohyoideus m.

Shaft of
mandible

Br. facial a. and v.

Digastricus m.

Platysma m.

Inferior labial
a. and v.

B

Approach to the Caudal Shaft and Ramus of the Mandible

INDICATION

Open reduction of fractures in this region.

ALTERNATIVE/COMBINATION APPROACHES

Plates 6 and 8

DESCRIPTION OF THE PROCEDURE

A. With the dog in dorsal recumbency, the incision is centered on the ventral surface of the mandible, extending from the angular process of the mandible cranially, approximately one half the length of the mandible.

B. The platysma muscle is incised with the skin to reveal the superficial portion of the masseter muscle laterally and the digastricus muscle lying ventromedially over the shaft of the mandible. An incision is made in the intermuscular septum between the masseter and the digastricus muscle. Lateral to this incision is the large facial vein and accompanying nerve trunks. The periosteal insertion of the digastricus muscle on the shaft of the mandible is incised and elevated.

C. Lateral retraction of the masseter and subperiosteal elevation of part of its insertion in the masseteric fossa allow good exposure of the lateral side of the shaft and ventral part of the ramus, and medial retraction of the digastricus and deeper lying mylohyoideus muscle gives exposure of the medial side of the shaft. The myelohyoideus and rostral insertion of the masseter muscle both can be elevated for more exposure of the ventral border of the mandible.

CLOSURE

The intermuscular septum between the digastricus and masseter muscles is closed, care being taken not to impinge the facial vessels. Platysma muscle is included with subcutaneous fascia in a separate layer.

Plate 7

Approach to the Caudal Shaft and Ramus of the Mandible

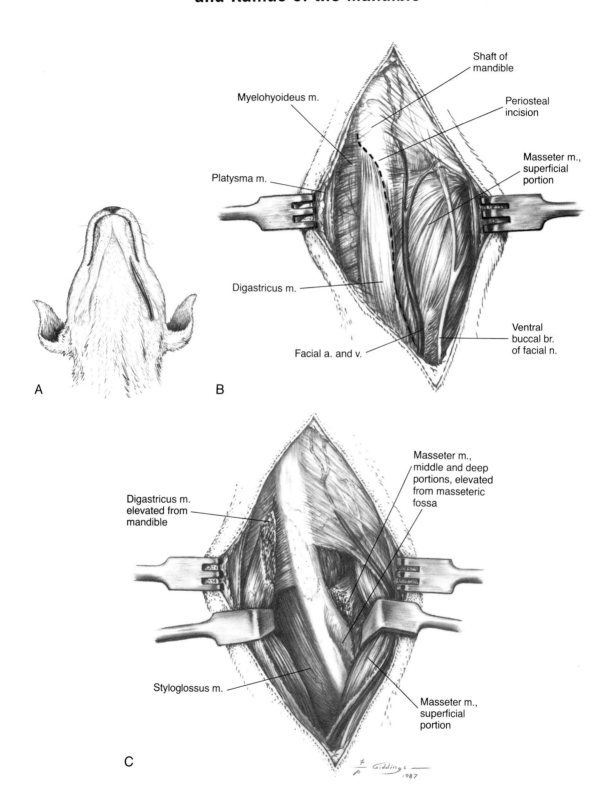

Shaft of mandible

Periosteal incision

Myelohyoideus m.

Masseter m., superficial portion

Platysma m.

Digastricus m.

Facial a. and v.

Ventral buccal br. of facial n.

A

B

Digastricus m. elevated from mandible

Masseter m., middle and deep portions, elevated from masseteric fossa

Styloglossus m.

Masseter m., superficial portion

C

Approach to the Ramus of the Mandible

INDICATION

Open reduction of fractures.

ALTERNATIVE/COMBINATION APPROACHES

Plates 7 and 9

DESCRIPTION OF THE PROCEDURE

A. The skin incision starts dorsally over the temporomandibular joint and extends rostroventrad to end over the mandibular shaft at the level of the last molar.

B. The incision is deepened through subcutaneous tissue and platysma muscle. The dorsal and ventral buccal branches of the facial nerve and the parotid gland and duct are identified and preserved. An incision is made across the fibers of the superficial layers of the masseter muscle, roughly paralleling the caudal border of the mandible.

C. After cutting through the superficial layer of the masseter muscle, the middle and deep layers can be elevated from their insertion on the caudal and ventral parts of the masseteric fossa. Careful dorsal dissection and retraction allow exposure of the ramus to the level of the temporomandibular joint.

CLOSURE

The middle and deep layers of the masseter muscle fall back against the mandible when the superficial layer incision is closed. Horizontal mattress sutures are placed in the strong aponeurosis covering the superficial layer of the masseter muscle. Platysma muscle and skin are closed in separate layers.

Plate 8

Approach to the Ramus of the Mandible

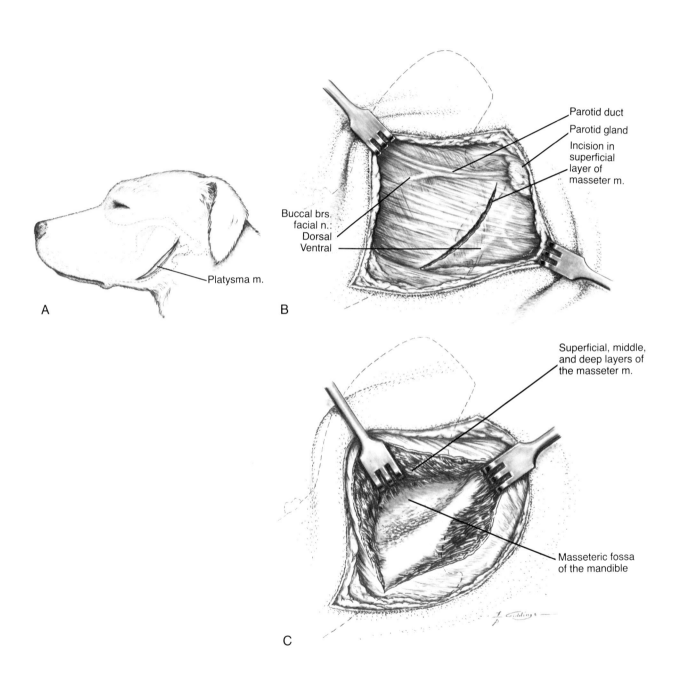

Platysma m.

A

Parotid duct
Parotid gland
Incision in
superficial
layer of
masseter m.

Buccal brs.
facial n.:
Dorsal
Ventral

B

Superficial, middle,
and deep layers of
the masseter m.

Masseteric fossa
of the mandible

C

Approach to the Temporomandibular Joint

INDICATIONS

1. Open reduction of luxations.
2. Open reduction of fractures.

ALTERNATIVE/COMBINATION APPROACH

Plate 8

DESCRIPTION OF THE PROCEDURE

A. The skin incision follows the ventral border of the zygomatic arch and crosses the temporomandibular joint caudally.

B. The platysma muscle, directly under the skin, is incised on the same line. A periosteal incision is made along the origin of the masseter muscle on the zygomatic arch.

C. Subperiosteal elevation of the masseter muscle exposes the joint. The mandibular condyle and interior of the joint are brought into view by wide incision of the joint capsule.

CLOSURE

The masseter muscle is sutured to fascia on the dorsal edge of the zygomatic arch. Platysma and skin are closed in separate layers.

Plate 9

Approach to the Temporomandibular Joint

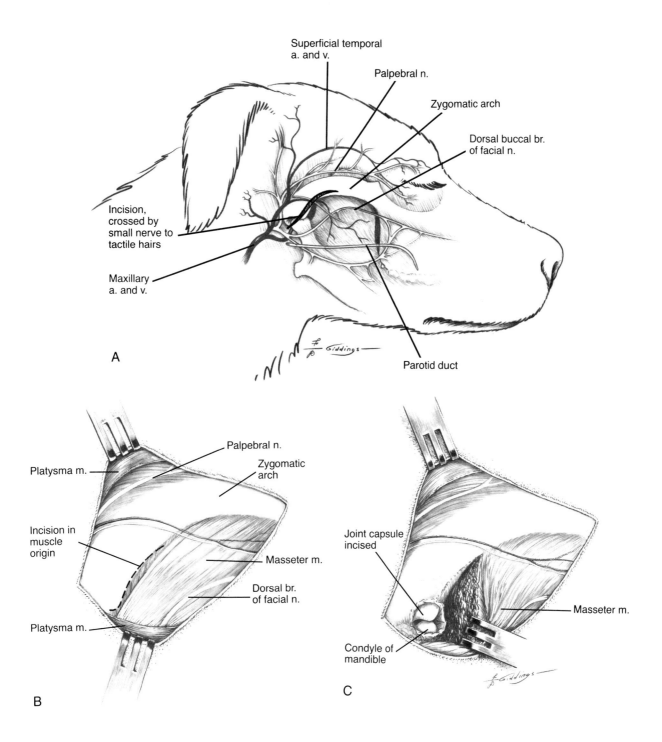

A

Superficial temporal a. and v.

Palpebral n.

Zygomatic arch

Dorsal buccal br. of facial n.

Incision, crossed by small nerve to tactile hairs

Maxillary a. and v.

Parotid duct

B

Platysma m.

Palpebral n.

Zygomatic arch

Incision in muscle origin

Masseter m.

Dorsal br. of facial n.

Platysma m.

C

Joint capsule incised

Masseter m.

Condyle of mandible

Approach to the Dorsolateral Surface of the Skull

Based on a Procedure of Hoerlein, Few, and Petty[14]

INDICATIONS

1. Open reduction of fractures of the frontal and parietal bones and the dorsal parts of the sphenoid and temporal bones.
2. Exposure of cerebral hemispheres.

DESCRIPTION OF THE PROCEDURE

A. The midline skin incision extends from the external occipital protuberance to the level of the eyes. Alternate incisions are also shown and are superior for reaching the more basilar area of the skull.

B. As the subcutaneous fascia is incised and retracted, three muscles are immediately encountered. Rostrally, these are the frontalis and interscutularis, the fibers of which run transversely, and caudally, the occipitalis with its fibers running parallel to the midline. These muscles are incised on the midline and retracted with the skin.

C. The temporalis muscle is covered by a layer of dense fascia, which is incised on the lateral side of the sagittal and frontal crests. The incision is then deepened to include the periosteum. One or both sides are incised, depending on the type of exposure desired.

D. The temporalis is elevated from the skull subperiosteally and retracted laterally. For bilateral exposure, both muscles are elevated and retracted.

CLOSURE

The temporal fascia is joined at the midline along the sagittal crest. Because the incisions curve laterally to follow the frontal crests, the temporal fascia is sutured to the loose fascia lying between the frontal crests. The frontalis, interscutularis, and occipitalis muscles are closed on the midline.

Plate 10

Approach to the Dorsolateral Surface of the Skull

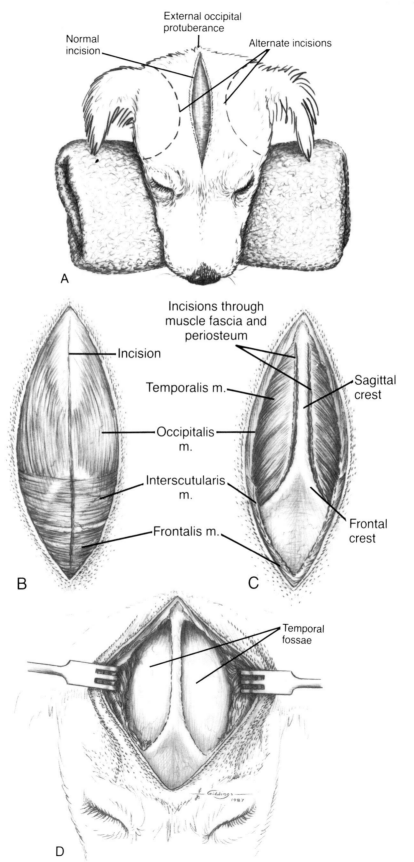

A

External occipital protuberance

Normal incision

Alternate incisions

Incisions through muscle fascia and periosteum

B

Incision

Temporalis m.

Occipitalis m.

Interscutularis m.

Frontalis m.

C

Sagittal crest

Frontal crest

D

Temporal fossae

Approach to the Caudal Surface of the Skull

Based on a Procedure of Hoerlein, Few, and Petty [14]

INDICATIONS

1. Open reduction of fractures of the occipital bone.
2. Exposure of the caudal portion of the cerebellum and the cranial portion of the brain stem.

DESCRIPTION OF THE PROCEDURE

A. The midline portion of the skin incision extends caudally from the external occipital protuberance to the spinous process of the axis (C2). The transverse incision follows the nuchal crest of the occiput and ends just short of the base of the ears.

   The subcutaneous fascia is incised in the same lines as the skin and is undermined with the skin to allow lateral retraction of each skin flap. The platysma muscle will be incised and retracted with subcutaneous fascia.

B. The first muscles seen upon retraction of the skin are the cervicoscutularis and superficial cervicoauricularis. Originating on the exposed area of the cervical midline and passing cranially toward the ears, these muscles resemble a chevron with the point situated caudally. The muscles are incised on the midline and each muscle belly allowed to retract. The temporal muscles, the external occipital protuberance, and the dorsal cervical muscles inserting on the occiput can now be visualized.

C. The splenius capitis and rhomboideus muscles are transected close to their origin on the nuchal line of the occiput. The use of electrocautery for this cutting is very helpful in minimizing hemorrhage. Enough tissue is left on the occiput to allow resuturing of the muscles. The midline incision runs from the external occipital protuberance to the spinous process of the axis (C2).

D. Muscle elevation continues laterally and ventrally to expose the occipital bone, the foramen magnum, and the dorsal arch of the atlas (C1).

CLOSURE

The cervical muscles are attached to the occiput by using mattress sutures that engage the fibrous muscle insertions remaining on the bone. The external sheath of the temporal muscles may also be used to securely anchor these sutures.

COMMENTS

The caudal brain stem and cranial spinal cord may be exposed by elevating the muscles from the atlas and performing a dorsal laminectomy on this vertebra.

Plate 11
Approach to the Caudal Surface of the Skull

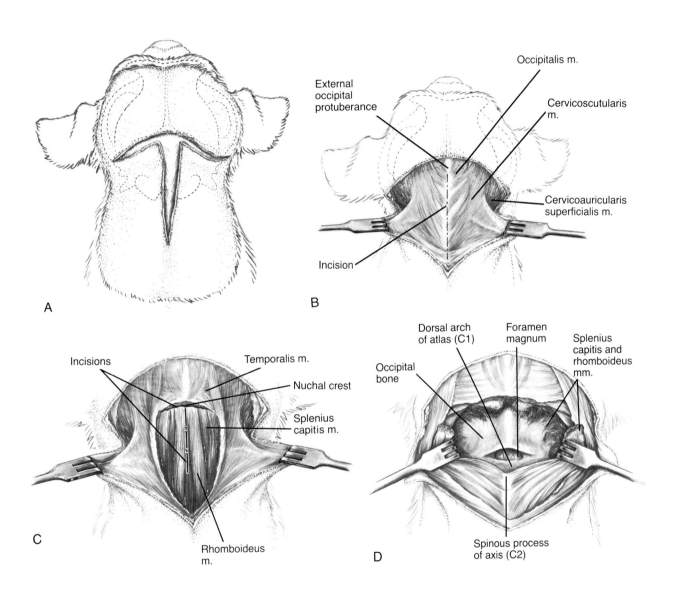

A

B

External occipital protuberance

Occipitalis m.

Cervicoscutularis m.

Cervicoauricularis superficialis m.

Incision

C

Incisions

Temporalis m.

Nuchal crest

Splenius capitis m.

Rhomboideus m.

D

Dorsal arch of atlas (C1)

Foramen magnum

Occipital bone

Splenius capitis and rhomboideus mm.

Spinous process of axis (C2)

The Vertebral Column

- Approach to Cervical Vertebrae 1 and 2 Through a Ventral Incision

- Approach to Cervical Vertebrae 1 and 2 Through a Dorsal Incision

- Approach to Cervical Vertebrae and Intervertebral Disks 2–7 Through a Ventral Incision

- Approach to the Midcervical Vertebrae Through a Dorsal Incision

- Approach to the Caudal Cervical and Cranial Thoracic Vertebrae Through a Dorsal Incision

- Approach to the Thoracolumbar Vertebrae Through a Dorsal Incision

- Approach to the Thoracolumbar Intervertebral Disks Through a Dorsolateral Incision

- Approach to the Thoracolumbar Intervertebral Disks Through a Lateral Incision

- Approach to Lumbar Vertebra 7 and the Sacrum Through a Dorsal Incision

- Approach to the Caudal Vertebrae Through a Dorsal Incision

Approach to Cervical Vertebrae 1 and 2 Through a Ventral Incision

Based on a procedure of Sorjonen and Shires [38]

INDICATIONS

1. Treatment of fractures of the ventral aspect of cervical vertebrae 1 and 2.
2. Arthrodesis of C1–C2 articulation for atlantoaxial instability.

ALTERNATIVE/COMBINATION APPROACH

Plate 14

DESCRIPTION OF THE PROCEDURE

A. The animal is placed in the supine position with a sandbag under the neck to cause marked extension of the cranial cervical vertebrae. Placing the animal in a V-trough will elevate the shoulder region and increase the extension of the cervical spine. The skin incision begins on the midline between the angles of the mandible and ends in the midcervical region.

B. The incision is deepened through the subcutis and between the paired bellies of the sternohyoideus muscles to expose the trachea.

C. Retraction of the sternohyoideus muscles exposes the larynx and its muscles. The right sternothyroideus muscle is isolated and detached from its insertion on the thyroid process of the larynx. The thyroid gland should be protected during this dissection.

Plate 12

Approach to Cervical Vertebrae 1 and 2
Through a Ventral Incision

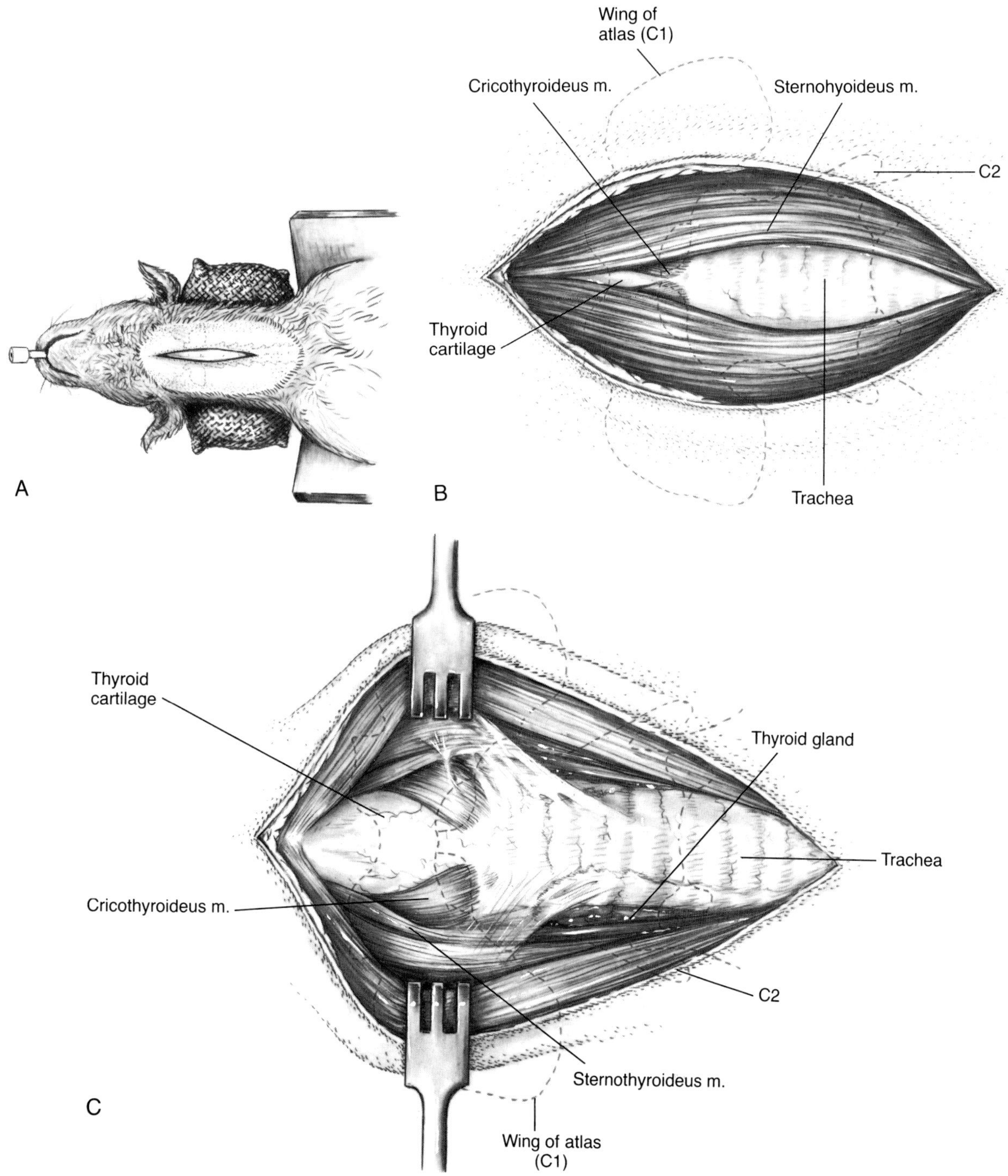

A

B

Wing of atlas (C1)

Cricothyroideus m.

Sternohyoideus m.

C2

Thyroid cartilage

Trachea

C

Thyroid cartilage

Thyroid gland

Trachea

Cricothyroideus m.

C2

Sternothyroideus m.

Wing of atlas (C1)

Approach to Cervical Vertebrae 1 and 2 Through a Ventral Incision *continued*

DESCRIPTION OF THE PROCEDURE *continued*

D. Retraction of the larynx and trachea to the left side (medially) is preceded by ligation or cautery of several small vessels running between the carotid artery/ internal jugular vein and the thyroid gland or trachea. The recurrent laryngeal nerve must be protected during this dissection and retraction. Muscle retraction to the right side (laterally) also includes the carotid artery, the internal jugular vein, and the vagosympathetic trunk. The longus colli muscles are now exposed. The ventral tubercle of C1 is located by palpation, and the longus colli muscle fibers are transected close to the tubercle.

E. Elevation of muscle fibers from the ventral arch of C1 and the body of C2 proceeds laterally until the articulations are exposed.

CLOSURE

Neither the deep fascia in the region of the trachea nor the longus colli muscles are sutured. The sternothyroideus muscle is reattached to the thyroid process by sutures, and the sternohyoideus muscles and subcutis are closed on the midline in layers.

Plate 12

Approach to Cervical Vertebrae 1 and 2 Through a Ventral Incision *continued*

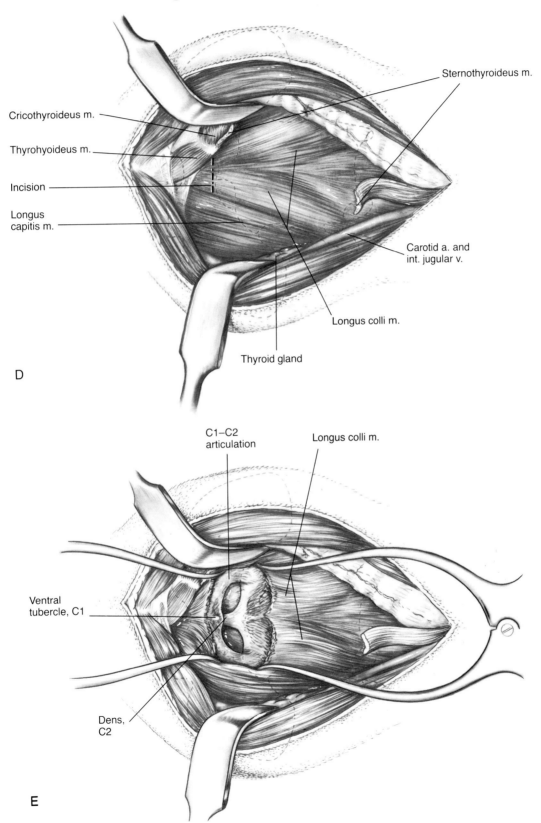

Cricothyroideus m.

Thyrohyoideus m.

Incision

Longus capitis m.

Sternothyroideus m.

Carotid a. and int. jugular v.

Longus colli m.

Thyroid gland

D

C1–C2 articulation

Longus colli m.

Ventral tubercle, C1

Dens, C2

E

Approach to Cervical Vertebrae 1 and 2 Through a Dorsal Incision

Based on a Procedure of Funkquist[11]

INDICATIONS

1. Open reduction of atlantoaxial luxation.
2. Open reduction of fractures of vertebrae C1 and C2.

ALTERNATIVE/COMBINATION APPROACHES

Plates 15 and 16

DESCRIPTION OF THE PROCEDURE

A. The skin incision is made on the dorsal midline starting at the level of the occipital protuberance, extending caudally to the level of the third or fourth cervical vertebra.

B. Skin is undermined and retracted and subcutaneous fascia incised on the midline to expose the occipitalis, cervicoscutularis, and cervicoauricularis superficialis muscles. Caudal and lateral to these muscles are the thin fibers of the platysma muscle. These muscles are incised on the midline fibrous raphe to allow elevation and lateral retraction of these muscles.

Plate 13
Approach to Cervical Vertebrae 1 and 2
Through a Dorsal Incision

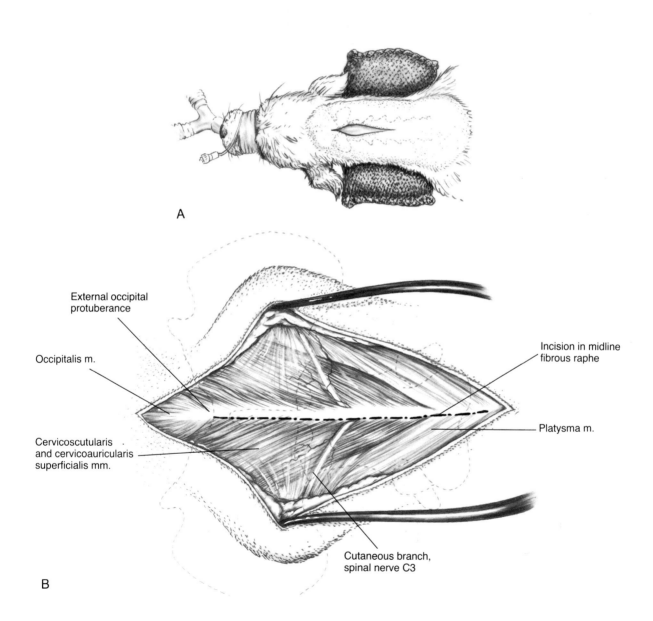

A

External occipital
protuberance

Occipitalis m.

Cervicoscutularis
and cervicoauricularis
superficialis mm.

Incision in midline
fibrous raphe

Platysma m.

Cutaneous branch,
spinal nerve C3

B

Approach to Cervical Vertebrae 1 and 2 Through a Dorsal Incision *continued*

DESCRIPTION OF THE PROCEDURE *continued*

C. Deepening the midline incision will allow separation of the paired bellies of the biventer cervicis superficially and the deeper rectus capitis attached to the dorsal spine of C2. The insertion of the rectus capitis muscle is incised along the lateral border of the spine of C2 to allow its elevation from the bone by combined sharp and blunt dissection.

D. As the dissection is carried deeper onto the lamina of C2, care should be taken to avoid the vertebral artery, which courses through the muscles slightly ventrolateral to the articular processes. The interarcuate (yellow) ligament covering the foramina between C1 and C2 is carefully incised to expose the spinal cord and the root of spinal nerve C1. The interarcuate of the foramen magnum may also be incised to expose the cranial rim of the dorsal arch of C1.

CLOSURE

Each muscle layer is closed on the midline to its opposite member.

COMMENTS

This exposure may be done bilaterally, using the same technique, where exposure of the entire dorsal aspect of the vertebrae is desirable.

Plate 13

Approach to Cervical Vertebrae 1 and 2
Through a Dorsal Incision *continued*

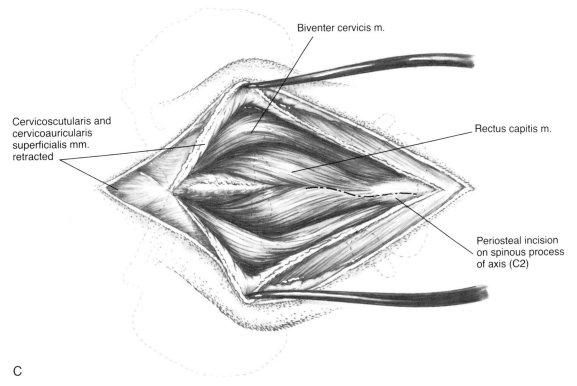

Biventer cervicis m.

Cervicoscutularis and
cervicoauricularis
superficialis mm.
retracted

Rectus capitis m.

Periosteal incision
on spinous process
of axis (C2)

C

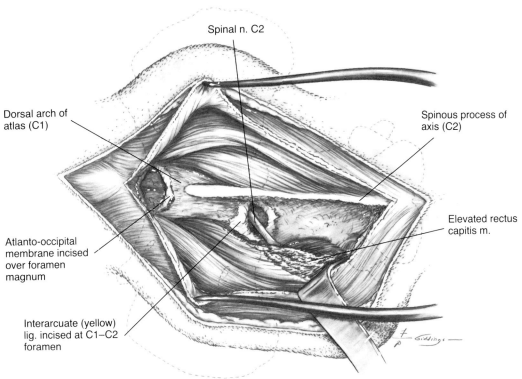

Spinal n. C2

Dorsal arch of
atlas (C1)

Spinous process of
axis (C2)

Atlanto-occipital
membrane incised
over foramen
magnum

Elevated rectus
capitis m.

Interarcuate (yellow)
lig. incised at C1–C2
foramen

D

Approach to Cervical Vertebrae and Intervertebral Disks 2–7 Through a Ventral Incision

Based on a Procedure of Olsson[26]

INDICATION

Fenestration and curettage of intervertebral disks C2–C7.

ALTERNATIVE/COMBINATION APPROACH

Plate 12

DESCRIPTION OF THE PROCEDURE

A. The animal, with tracheal catheter in place, is secured in the supine position. A sandbag is placed under the neck to cause definite extension of the cervical vertebral column. It is often useful to elevate the body by positioning the animal's trunk in a V-shaped trough, in order to gain more extension of the cervical spine. The skin incision extends from the manubrium to the larynx.

B. The incision is deepened by midline separation of the paired bellies of the mastoid part of the sternocephalicus muscle and underlying sternohyoideus muscle.

C. Lateral retraction of these muscles exposes the trachea, esophagus, deep cervical fascia, carotid sheath, and internal jugular vein.

Plate 14

Approach to Cervical Vertebrae and Intervertebral Disks 2–7 Through a Ventral Incision

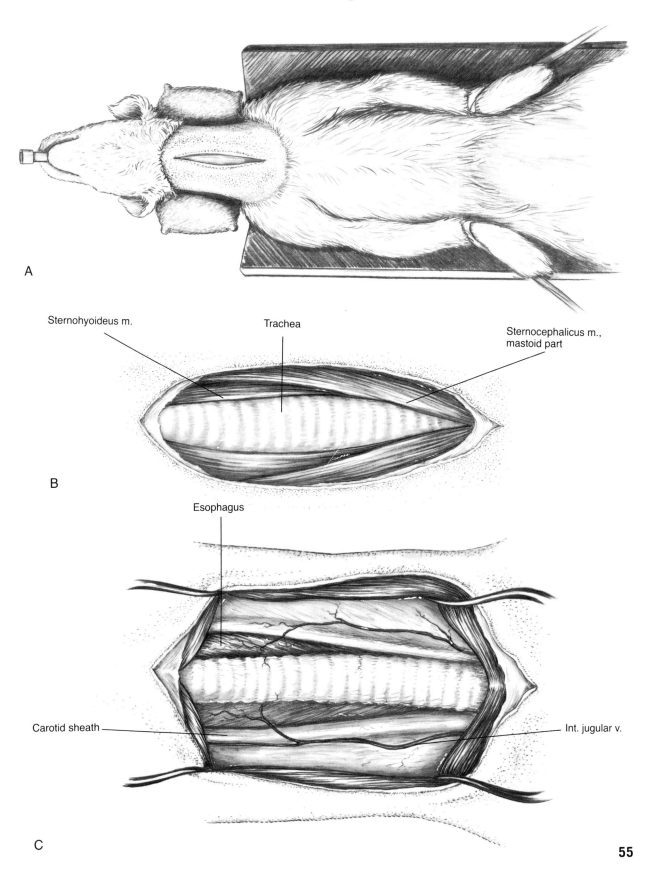

A

Sternohyoideus m.

Trachea

Sternocephalicus m., mastoid part

B

Esophagus

Carotid sheath

Int. jugular v.

C

Approach to Cervical Vertebrae and Intervertebral Disks 2–7 Through a Ventral Incision *continued*

DESCRIPTION OF THE PROCEDURE *continued*

D. Left lateral retraction of the trachea and esophagus allows blunt dissection close to the trachea, taking care not to injure the recurrent laryngeal nerve, through the deep cervical fascia to the longus colli muscle, which covers the ventral surfaces of the cervical vertebrae. The midline ventral crest of the vertebrae can be palpated through this muscle. A short transverse incision is made through the longus colli tendon of insertion just caudal to the crest.

E. Separation of longus colli muscle fibers overlying each ventral crest exposes the disk.

Plate 14

Approach to Cervical Vertebrae and Intervertebral Disks 2–7 Through a Ventral Incision *continued*

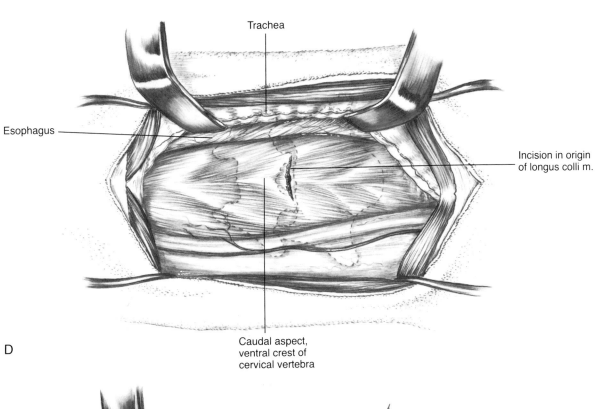

Trachea

Esophagus

Incision in origin of longus colli m.

Caudal aspect, ventral crest of cervical vertebra

D

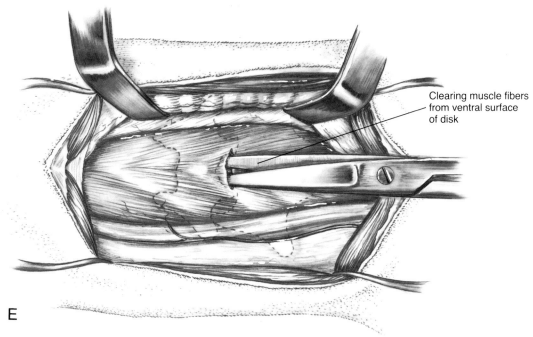

Clearing muscle fibers from ventral surface of disk

E

Approach to Cervical Vertebrae and Intervertebral Disks 2–7 Through a Ventral Incision *continued*

F. By working caudally from the prominence, the tendon is gently scraped from the bone until the ventral longitudinal ligament is exposed. The exact location of the intervertebral space can be identified by exploration with a 22-gauge needle, which is walked off the crest caudally until it penetrates the ventral longitudinal ligament and the annulus fibrosus of the disk.

G. Fenestration is accomplished by a stab incision through the ventral longitudinal ligament and the annulus fibrosus. This opening into the disk may have to be enlarged for disk curettage.

CLOSURE

The deep fascia is not sutured. The sternohyoideus and mastoid part of the sternocephalicus muscle are closed along the midline, and the subcutaneous fascia is likewise united.

COMMENTS

Care must be used in the retraction of tissues to avoid damage to the carotid sheath, the esophagus and trachea, and the right recurrent laryngeal nerve, which lies on the right dorsolateral aspect of the trachea. The location of a specific intervertebral space is determined by first identifying the caudal borders of the wings of the atlas by palpation. The ventral midline crest that lies on a line directly between the wings is the ventral tubercle of the atlas (C1). Other vertebrae can then be numbered by counting caudally from C1. Alternatively, the large transverse processes of C6 are easily palpated. The C5–C6 disk is between and slightly cranial to the cranial edges of the processes.

Plate 14

Approach to Cervical Vertebrae and Intervertebral Disks 2–7 Through a Ventral Incision *continued*

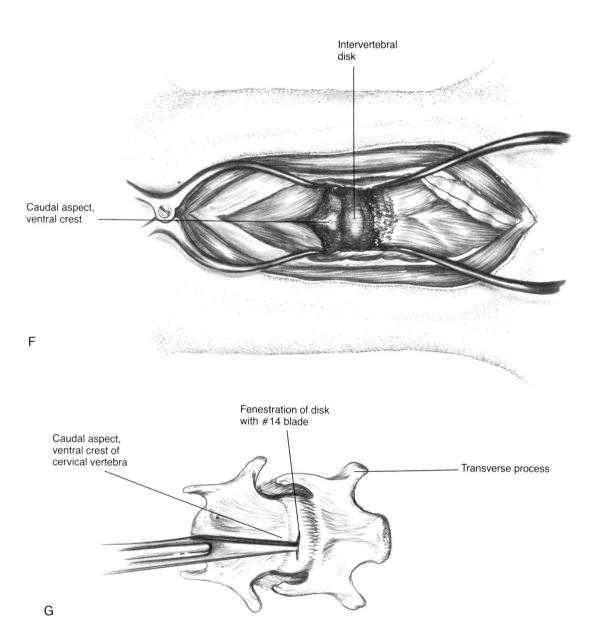

Intervertebral disk

Caudal aspect, ventral crest

F

Fenestration of disk with #14 blade

Caudal aspect, ventral crest of cervical vertebra

Transverse process

G

Approach to the Midcervical Vertebrae Through a Dorsal Incision

Based on a Procedure of Funkquist[11]

INDICATIONS

1. Open reduction of fractures and luxations of vertebrae C2–C5.
2. Dorsal laminectomy of vertebrae C2–C5.

ALTERNATIVE/COMBINATION APPROACHES

Plates 13 and 16

DESCRIPTION OF THE PROCEDURE

A. The animal is positioned in sternal recumbency, with a sandbag placed under the neck to elevate it and to cause flexion of the cervical spine. A tracheal catheter is imperative to maintain a patent airway in this position.

 The midline skin incision extends from the external occipital protuberance to the first thoracic vertebra.

B. As the subcutaneous fascia is incised and the skin margins retracted, the almost transparent fibrous aponeurosis of the platysma muscle comes into view.

 An incision is now made through the median fibrous raphe. This incision is deepened until the nuchal ligament (missing in the cat) is exposed.

Plate 15

Approach to the Midcervical Vertebrae Through a Dorsal Incision

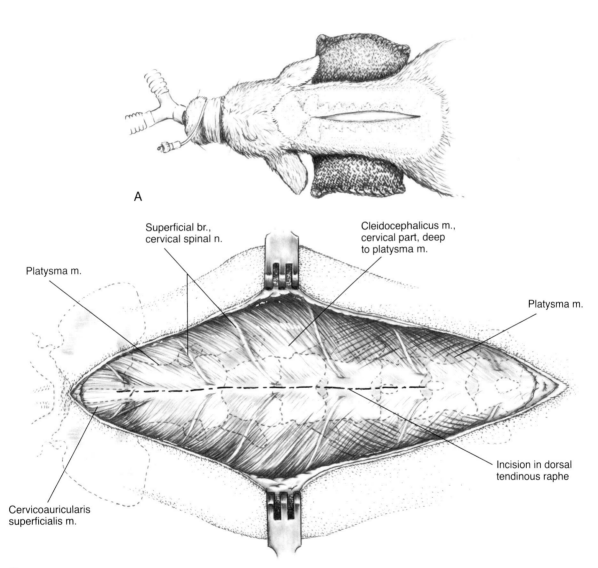

A

Platysma m.

Superficial br.,
cervical spinal n.

Cleidocephalicus m.,
cervical part, deep
to platysma m.

Platysma m.

Incision in dorsal
tendinous raphe

Cervicoauricularis
superficialis m.

B

Approach to the Midcervical Vertebrae Through a Dorsal
Incision *continued*

DESCRIPTION OF THE PROCEDURE *continued*

C. The dorsolateral cervical muscles separated by this incision are retracted laterally to expose the nuchal ligament. The spinous processes can now be palpated under the ligament.

   An incision is made in the rectus capitis, spinalis et semispinalis cervicis, and multifidus muscles along one side of the nuchal ligament. The incision is deepened along the lateral side of the spinous processes to the vertebral laminae.

D. Elevation with a periosteal elevator and retraction of the muscles from the vertebrae are done first on the side that was incised. The insertion of the nuchal ligament is now elevated from the spinous process of the axis, and the ligament is retracted with the muscles on the side opposite the incision. The ligament remains firmly attached to the muscles of one side and cranially to the axis.

   Lateral elevation of muscles from the laminae should be limited to the lateral aspect of the articular processes in order to avoid branches of the vertebral artery coursing ventrolaterally to the processes.

CLOSURE

The nuchal ligament is secured to the axis by two sutures of nonabsorbable material. These sutures are passed through holes drilled transversely through the spinous process of the axis.

The external fascia of the deep muscles can now be sutured to the nuchal ligament. The median fibrous raphe is closed next, followed by the subcutaneous fascia.

COMMENTS

If the spinous process of the axis has been removed in the course of laminectomy, the nuchal ligament is secured to the rectus capitis muscle by mattress sutures that bite deeply into this muscle.

Plate 15

Approach to the Midcervical Vertebrae
Through a Dorsal Incision *continued*

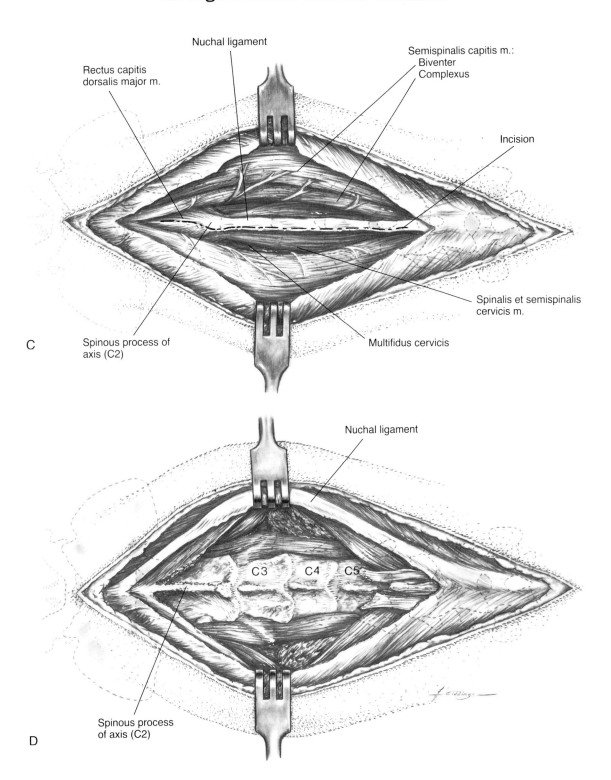

Nuchal ligament

Rectus capitis
dorsalis major m.

Semispinalis capitis m.:
Biventer
Complexus

Incision

Spinalis et semispinalis
cervicis m.

Spinous process of
axis (C2)

Multifidus cervicis

C

Nuchal ligament

C3   C4   C5

Spinous process
of axis (C2)

D

Approach to the Caudal Cervical and Cranial Thoracic Vertebrae Through a Dorsal Incision

Based on a Procedure of Parker[29]

INDICATIONS

1. Dorsal laminectomy for decompression of the spinal cord for ruptured intervertebral disk or vertebral fractures of C5 through T3.
2. Resection of tumors of the spinal cord or vertebral lamina and dorsal spines of C5 through T3.

ALTERNATIVE/COMBINATION APPROACHES

Plates 13, 15, and 17

DESCRIPTION OF THE PROCEDURE

A. With the animal in sternal recumbency, the forelegs are crossed under the chest and tied to the opposite sides of the table. Sandbags are useful to prevent shifting of position and to position the head, which can lie on the table. A skin incision is made on the dorsal midline from the midcervical to the cranial thoracic region, approximately C4 to T6.

B. The dorsal midline tendinous raphe is seen after incision of subcutaneous tissues on the midline. At this point a decision must be made as to which side of the midline will be chosen for the dissection. This may be dictated by pathology present or may be the choice of the surgeon. An incision is made in the tendinous raphe slightly toward the side selected (right side is illustrated).

Plate 16
Approach to the Caudal Cervical and Cranial Thoracic Vertebrae Through a Dorsal Incision

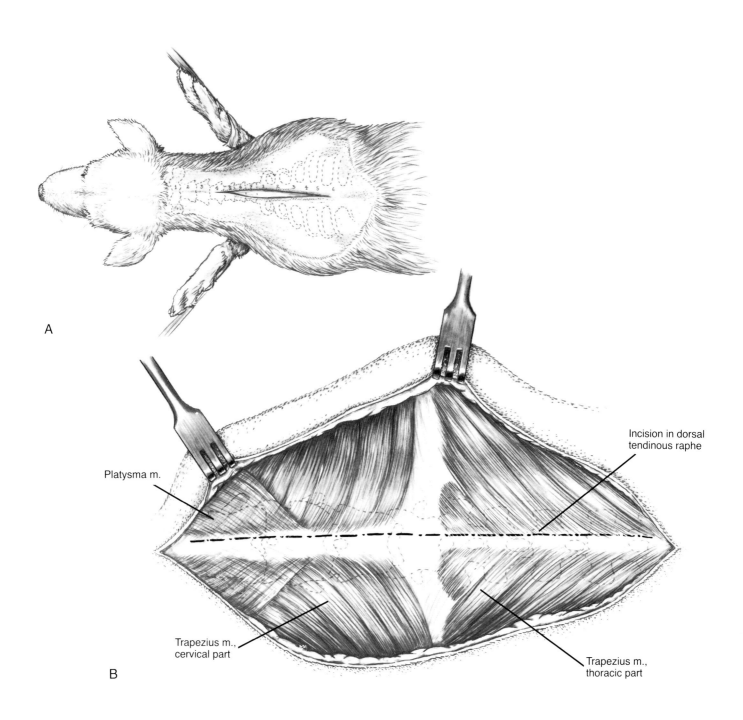

A

B

Incision in dorsal tendinous raphe

Platysma m.

Trapezius m., cervical part

Trapezius m., thoracic part

Approach to the Caudal Cervical and Cranial Thoracic Vertebrae Through a Dorsal Incision *continued*

DESCRIPTION OF THE PROCEDURE *continued*

C. Trapezius and rhomboideus muscles can be retracted to reveal the medial surface of the subscapularis muscle, the splenius muscle cranially, and the serratus dorsalis muscle caudally. The right scapula can now be retracted laterally. Incisions are now made in the origin of the splenius and the serratus dorsalis muscles on the tendinous raphe. A portion of the cranial serratus muscle may originate from fascia of the splenius.

Plate 16

Approach to the Caudal Cervical and Cranial Thoracic Vertebrae Through a Dorsal Incision *continued*

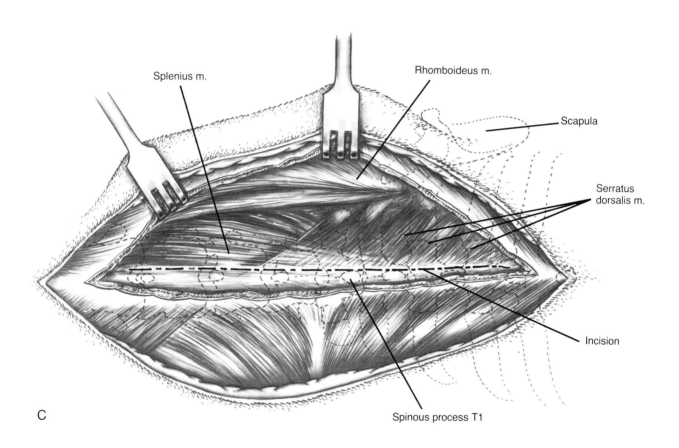

Splenius m.

Rhomboideus m.

Scapula

Serratus dorsalis m.

Incision

Spinous process T1

C

Approach to the Caudal Cervical and Cranial Thoracic Vertebrae Through a Dorsal Incision *continued*

DESCRIPTION OF THE PROCEDURE *continued*

D. Lateral retraction of the splenius and serratus dorsalis muscles exposes the nuchal ligament, the dorsal thoracic spines, and the underlying long spinal muscles. These muscles, the longissimus thoracis et lumborum, the spinalis et semispinalis thoracis, and the spinalis cervicis, are separated from the midline by a combination of sharp and blunt dissection. As this dissection proceeds ventrally along the lateral surfaces of the dorsal vertebral spines, the dorsal laminae of the vertebrae will come into view.

E. Continued dissection of the long spinal muscles and the multifidus muscle will completely expose the dorsal laminae and pedicles of the vertebrae. The surgeon must be aware of the danger of incising or tearing the vertebral artery ventral to the articular processes. This artery can be damaged when elevating muscle bellies from C7 and T1. Once torn, ligation is difficult and pressure must be used for hemostasis. The large interarcuate space between C7 and T1 can be palpated and the yellow ligament incised to expose the spinal cord. The size of this space makes it an ideal starting point for dorsal laminectomy, as does the space between C6–C7.

CLOSURE

All muscle bellies are attached to the midline tendinous raphe or nuchal ligament in layers. The considerable subcutaneous tissues merit special care in closure to prevent seroma formation.

COMMENTS

In order to perform a dorsal laminectomy, the dorsal spines of the affected vertebrae must be removed. This creates some apparent difficulty with the thoracic vertebrae, because the nuchal ligament originates on the spines of T1–T3. These spines can, however, be cut with no ill effects, because the nuchal ligament is somewhat continuous with the supraspinous ligament. This gives the effect of lengthening the nuchal ligament's origin caudal to the dorsal spine of T3.

Plate 16

Approach to the Caudal Cervical and Cranial Thoracic Vertebrae Through a Dorsal Incision *continued*

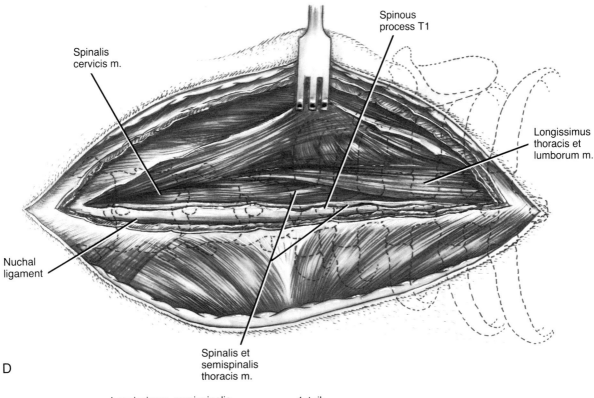

Spinous process T1

Spinalis cervicis m.

Longissimus thoracis et lumborum m.

Nuchal ligament

Spinalis et semispinalis thoracis m.

D

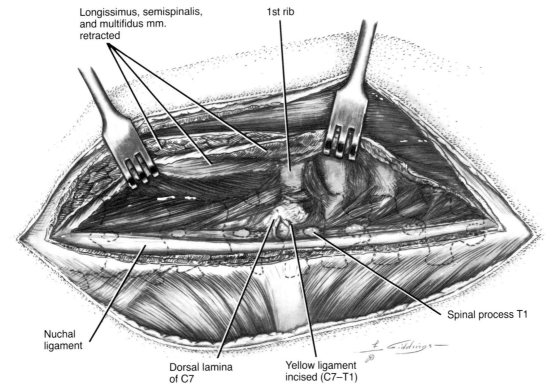

Longissimus, semispinalis, and multifidus mm. retracted

1st rib

Nuchal ligament

Dorsal lamina of C7

Yellow ligament incised (C7–T1)

Spinal process T1

E

Approach to the Thoracolumbar Vertebrae Through a Dorsal Incision

Based on a Procedure of Redding[31]

INDICATIONS

1. Open reduction of fractures and luxations of the vertebrae.
2. Dorsal laminectomy and hemilaminectomy.

ALTERNATIVE/COMBINATION APPROACHES

Plates 16, 18, and 20

EXPLANATORY NOTE

The exposure for hemilaminectomy is unilateral and is illustrated and described in A–E below. For laminectomy, a bilateral exposure is needed and is achieved by repeating steps B–E on the contralateral side. The final results are illustrated in Part F.

DESCRIPTION OF THE PROCEDURE

A. The length of the dorsal midline incision is determined by the number of vertebrae that are to be exposed. In order to obtain sufficient muscle retraction, it is necessary to extend the incision the length of two vertebrae cranial and caudal to the vertebra in question. The incision shown here centers on L1, extends from T12 to L3, and is made 5 to 10 mm from the midline.

B. Subcutaneous fat and fascia are incised until the dense lumbodorsal fascia is reached. The fat is undermined to free it from the fascia and to allow its retraction with the skin.

   The fascia and supraspinous ligament are incised around each spinous process and on the midline between each process. The incision is deepened to the laminae to complete the midline muscle separation.

Plate 17

Approach to the Thoracolumbar Vertebrae Through a Dorsal Incision

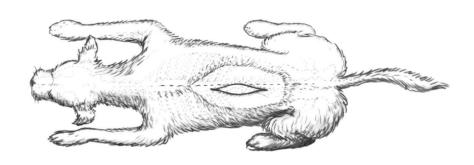

A

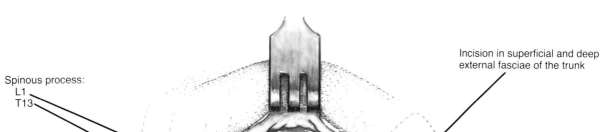

Spinous process:
L1
T13

Incision in superficial and deep
external fasciae of the trunk

B

Approach to the Thoracolumbar Vertebrae Through a Dorsal Incision *continued*

DESCRIPTION OF THE PROCEDURE *continued*

C. The multifidus lumborum muscle is sharply elevated from each spinous process and then bluntly elevated from the laminae laterally to the mamillary processes. This is sufficient exposure for a dorsal laminectomy when done bilaterally. Elevation is most easily done from a caudal-to-cranial direction. See Part F.

D. For hemilaminectomy, the multifidus must be incised and freed from the mamillary processes. The incision should be made directly on the bone to limit hemorrhage, and the underlying dorsal nerve root and vessels must be protected.

Plate 17

Approach to the Thoracolumbar Vertebrae
Through a Dorsal Incision *continued*

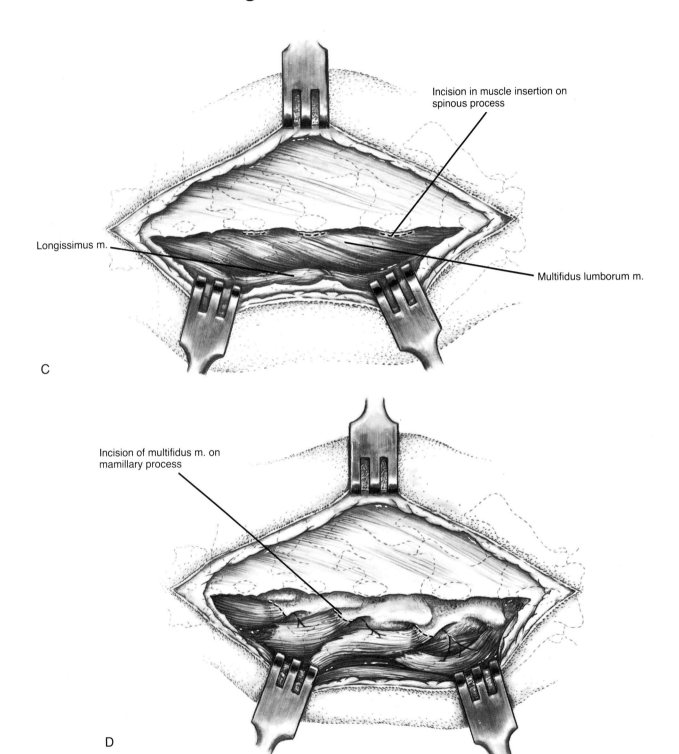

Incision in muscle insertion on
spinous process

Longissimus m.

Multifidus lumborum m.

C

Incision of multifidus m. on
mamillary process

D

Approach to the Thoracolumbar Vertebrae Through a Dorsal Incision *continued*

DESCRIPTION OF THE PROCEDURE *continued*

E. Lateral retraction of the muscles exposes the mamillary processes, nerve roots and vessels, and the rib head or transverse processes.

F. The exposure as done for laminectomy. Compare to Part D.

CLOSURE

The lumbodorsal fascia is sutured at the dorsal midline. The subcutaneous fat and fascia are closed with a second layer of sutures, followed by closure of the skin.

Plate 17

Approach to the Thoracolumbar Vertebrae
Through a Dorsal Incision *continued*

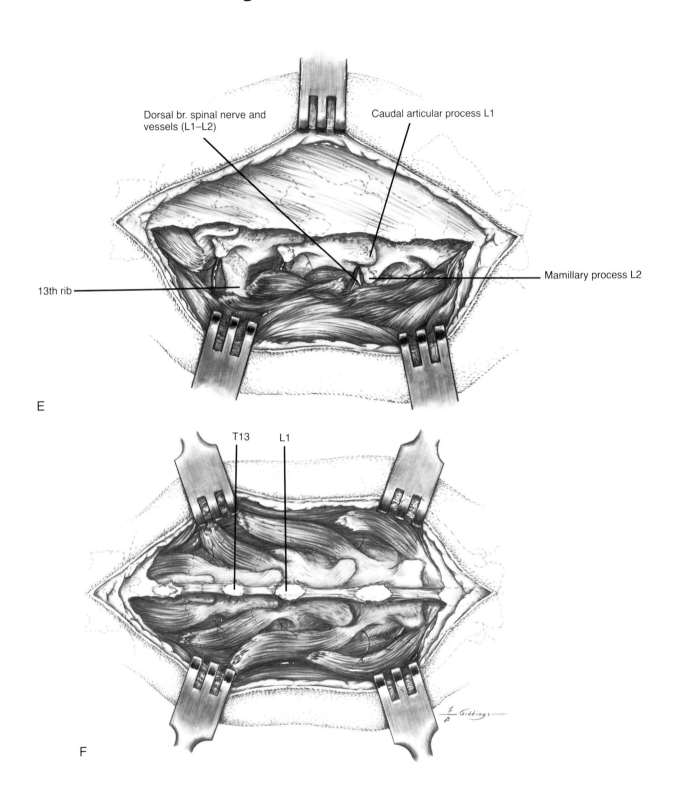

Dorsal br. spinal nerve and vessels (L1–L2)

Caudal articular process L1

13th rib

Mamillary process L2

E

T13   L1

F

Approach to the Thoracolumbar Intervertebral Disks Through a Dorsolateral Incision

Based on a Procedure of Yturraspe and Lumb[43]

INDICATION

Fenestration and curettage of intervertebral disks T10 through L5.

ALTERNATIVE/COMBINATION APPROACH

Plate 19

DESCRIPTION OF THE PROCEDURE

A. The dog is positioned in ventral recumbency with the hindlimbs flexed to maintain the normal curvative of the spine. The skin incision is made slightly to the left side of the midline for a right-handed surgeon. A left-handed surgeon should operate from the dog's right side. The incision extends from the eighth thoracic to the seventh lumbar vertebra.

B. Subcutaneous fat is elevated from the deep fascia of the trunk for a distance of 1.5 cm lateral to the dorsal spinous processes. This exposes the spinalis et semispinalis muscle cranially and the superficial layer of the deep external fascia of the trunk caudally. Both the deep and superficial layers of this fascia originate on the dorsal spinous processes. Both layers of the fascia are incised 5 to 10 mm from the dorsal spines in the midlumbar area, and this incision is continued caudally to the limits of the skin incision. As the fascial incision approaches the spinalis et semispinalis muscle cranially, it is directed medially so that it ends only 1 to 2 mm lateral to the spinous processes. A portion of this muscle must be incised in order to extend the incision cranially over the ribs.

Plate 18

Approach to the Thoracolumbar Intervertebral Disks Through a Dorsolateral Incision

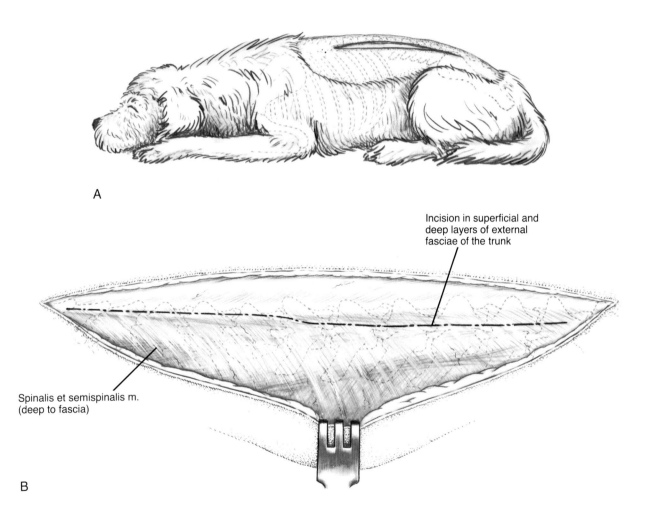

A

Incision in superficial and
deep layers of external
fasciae of the trunk

Spinalis et semispinalis m.
(deep to fascia)

B

Approach to the Thoracolumbar Intervertebral Disks Through a Dorsolateral Incision *continued*

DESCRIPTION OF THE PROCEDURE *continued*

C. The multifidus and longissimus muscles are separated by blunt dissection of the intermuscular septum. This septum is the first distinct muscle division lateral to the spinous processes and is most obvious in the midlumbar region. This separation is done with sweeping strokes with dissection scissors partially opened and directed in a craniomedial direction. Proceeding from caudal to cranial is advantageous during this dissection.

D. As the dissection deepens, small tendons will be encountered, crossing the dissection in a craniomedial direction, and they should be preserved. The tendons are attachments of the longissimus muscle to the accessory processes of the vertebrae. In the thoracic region, the tendon divides and attaches both to the rib and the accessory process. The dorsal branches of the spinal nerves emerge just ventral to these tendinous insertions, and the intervertebral disk space is located caudoventral to the insertions.

E. Exposure of disks is best done with a small curved periosteal elevator. Using the thirteenth rib as a landmark, the elevator is used to remove muscle and fascia overlying each disk. The insertions of the longissimus tendons are used as landmarks for locating the disk spaces. A nerve root retractor allows the spinal nerves to be retracted cranially and protected from the elevation and fenestrating instruments. T10–T11 is the most cranial disk accessible, and L5–L6 the most caudal.

CLOSURE

Both layers of the deep external fascia of the trunk are closed together. Subcutaneous fat and fascia and skin are closed in separate layers.

Plate 18

Approach to the Thoracolumbar Intervertebral Disks
Through a Dorsolateral Incision *continued*

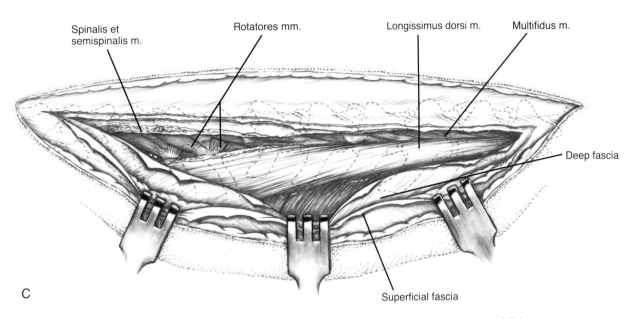

Spinalis et semispinalis m. — Rotatores mm. — Longissimus dorsi m. — Multifidus m. — Deep fascia — Superficial fascia

C

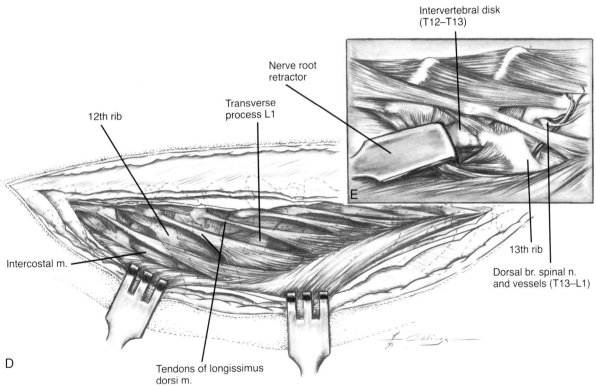

12th rib — Transverse process L1 — Nerve root retractor — Intervertebral disk (T12–T13) — 13th rib — Dorsal br. spinal n. and vessels (T13–L1) — Intercostal m. — Tendons of longissimus dorsi m. — E

D

Approach to the Thoracolumbar Intervertebral Disks Through a Lateral Incision

Based on Procedures of Flo and Brinker,[10] and Seeman[33]

INDICATION

Fenestration of thoracolumbar disks T10–L5.

ALTERNATIVE/COMBINATION APPROACH

Plate 18

DESCRIPTION OF THE PROCEDURE

A. The skin incision is slightly oblique, extending from the base of rib 10 toward the cranioventral iliac spine. The subcutaneous fat is usually quite thick here and is incised on the skin line to reveal the superficial thoracolumbar fascia.

B. The superficial thoracolumbar fascia is incised along the same line.

Plate 19

Approach to the Thoracolumbar Intervertebral Disks
Through a Lateral Incision

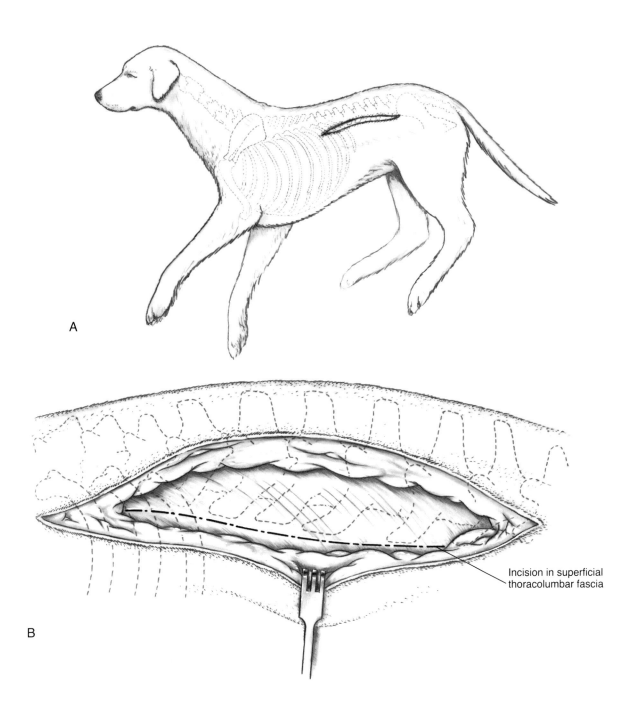

A

B

Incision in superficial
thoracolumbar fascia

Approach to the Thoracolumbar Intervertebral Disks Through a Lateral Incision *continued*

DESCRIPTION OF THE PROCEDURE *continued*

C. The deep thoracolumbar fascia is incised to reveal a second layer of fat and the underlying muscles. The lateral processes can now be palpated quite easily. To approach the thoracic spaces, it is necessary to transect some bundles of the serratus dorsalis muscle.

D. The thirteenth rib is a good place to start, because it allows counting cranially and caudally to identify the other vertebrae. Blunt dissection and separation of the fibers of the iliocostalis lumborum muscle allow the proximal end of the thirteenth rib to be exposed. A periosteal elevator is used to clear soft tissues from the cranial border of the rib and the lateral surface of the disk. Staying close to the cranial edge of the rib and strong cranial retraction of the muscle will protect the spinal nerve and vessel (see inset drawing). Care must be taken to prevent penetrating the thoracic pleura when clearing the disk surface.

   The lumbar disks are exposed by blunt separation of muscle tissue over the end of the appropriate lateral process. Confining the dissection and elevation to the dorsal surface of the process will protect vessels running along the cranial and caudal borders of the tip of the process. The elevation of muscle tissue is continued medially until the disk space is exposed. As the vertebral body and disk are approached, all elevation and retraction should be from a caudal-to-cranial direction to protect the spinal vessel and nerve. A blood vessel will be seen crossing the surface of the disk in the lower lumbar spaces, and it is usually lacerated during the fenestration process.

CLOSURE

The superficial and deep layers of the thoracolumbar fascia are closed with a continuous pattern and absorbable material. They can both be closed in one layer if the intervening fat is not too thick. Subcutaneous and skin layers are closed routinely.

COMMENTS

The choice between this approach and the dorsolateral approach (Plate 18) is a matter of personal choice. The exposure obtained is similar in both.

Plate 19

Approach to the Thoracolumbar Intervertebral Disks Through a Lateral Incision *continued*

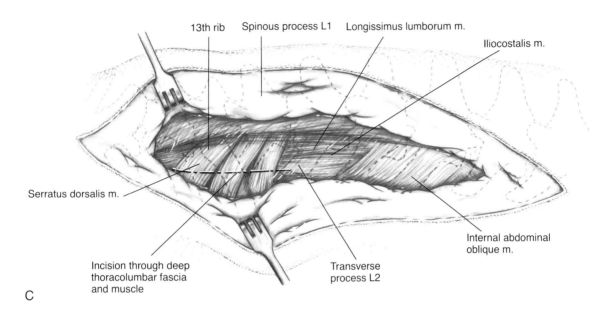

13th rib Spinous process L1 Longissimus lumborum m.

Iliocostalis m.

Serratus dorsalis m.

Incision through deep
thoracolumbar fascia
and muscle

Transverse
process L2

Internal abdominal
oblique m.

C

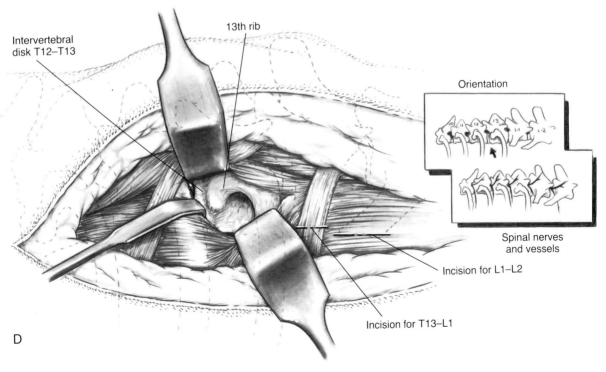

Intervertebral
disk T12–T13

13th rib

Orientation

Spinal nerves
and vessels

Incision for L1–L2

Incision for T13–L1

D

Approach to Lumbar Vertebra 7 and the Sacrum Through a Dorsal Incision

INDICATIONS

1. Laminectomy of L7–S1.
2. Open reduction of fractures of L7 or S1.

ALTERNATIVE/COMBINATION APPROACHES

Plates 17 and 21

DESCRIPTION OF THE PROCEDURE

A. A dorsal midline incision is made between the spine of the sixth lumbar vertebra and the caudal median sacral crest. Subcutaneous fat and superficial fascia are incised on the same line to expose the deep gluteal and caudal fasciae, which are also incised on the midline and around each spinous process.

B. The sacrocaudalis dorsal medialis muscles are freed from the spinous processes by incising around each process, then along the midline between processes. Elevation of the muscles is done with a sharp periosteal elevator, working from caudal to cranial.

Plate 20

Approach to Lumbar Vertebra 7 and the Sacrum
Through a Dorsal Incision

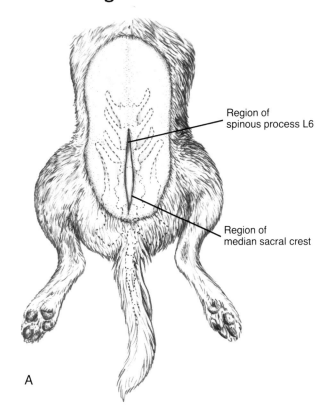

Region of
spinous process L6

Region of
median sacral crest

A

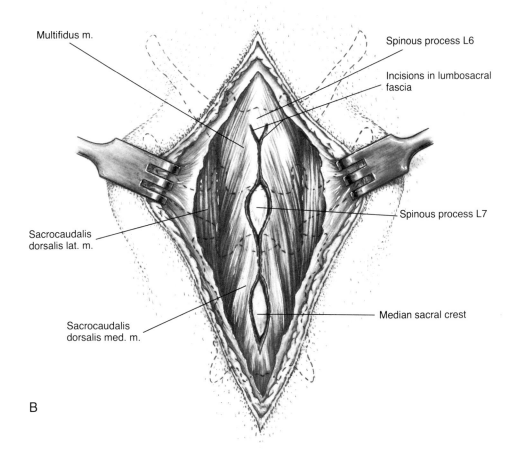

Multifidus m.

Spinous process L6

Incisions in lumbosacral
fascia

Spinous process L7

Sacrocaudalis
dorsalis lat. m.

Sacrocaudalis
dorsalis med. m.

Median sacral crest

B

Approach to Lumbar Vertebra 7 and the Sacrum Through a Dorsal Incision *continued*

DESCRIPTION OF THE PROCEDURE *continued*

C, D. Muscle elevation is continued laterally to the region of L6–L7 and L7–S1 articular processes cranially and to the intermediate sacral crests caudally. Just lateral to the crests are the dorsal sacral foramina, through which pass the dorsal branches of the sacral nerves and vessels. The interarcuate (yellow) ligament between the laminae of L7–S1 is incised to expose the cauda equina nerves.

CLOSURE

The gluteal and caudal fasciae are closed on the midline. Because of its considerable depth, the subcutaneous fat may need to be closed in two layers.

Plate 20

Approach to Lumbar Vertebra 7 and the Sacrum Through a Dorsal Incision *continued*

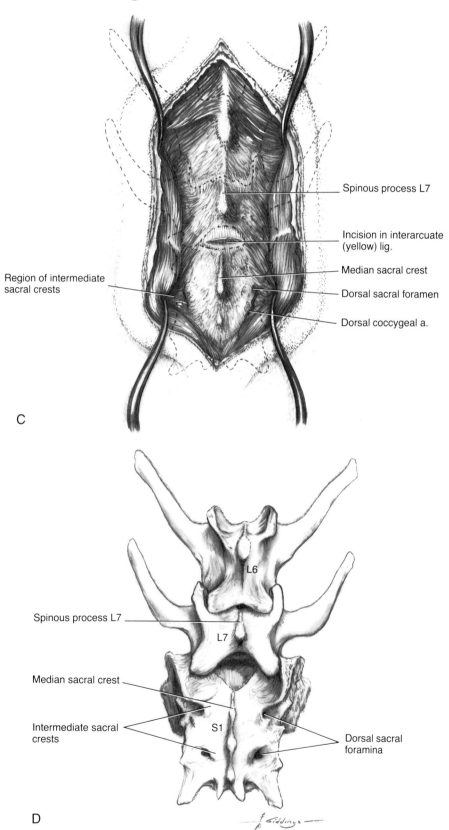

Spinous process L7

Incision in interarcuate (yellow) lig.

Median sacral crest

Region of intermediate sacral crests

Dorsal sacral foramen

Dorsal coccygeal a.

C

L6

Spinous process L7

L7

Median sacral crest

Intermediate sacral crests

S1

Dorsal sacral foramina

D

Approach to the Caudal Vertebrae Through a Dorsal Incision

INDICATIONS

1. Open reduction of fractures and luxations of the caudal vertebrae.
2. Treatment of malunion fractures or congenital malformation of the vertebrae by osteotomy.

ALTERNATIVE/COMBINATION APPROACH

Plate 20

DESCRIPTION OF THE PROCEDURE

A. The skin and subcutaneous fascial incision is made along the dorsal midline of the tail and extends the length of one vertebra proximal and distal to the vertebra to be exposed.

B. Undermining and retraction of the skin margins reveal the sacrocaudalis muscles under a layer of deep caudal fascia. This fascia is incised on the midline between the paired medial sacrocaudalis dorsalis muscles. The incision is continued into the intermuscular septum, until the dorsal surfaces of the vertebrae are reached.

C. A combination of sharp and blunt dissection is used to elevate the muscles from the vertebrae.

D. Only by working close to the bone during the muscular elevation can the dorsal lateral caudal arteries and nerves be avoided.

CLOSURE

Deep and subcutaneous fasciae are closed in one layer of sutures, followed by closure of the skin.

COMMENTS

The tail should be bandaged to minimize movement as much as possible for 5 to 7 days postoperatively.

Plate 21

Approach to the Caudal Vertebrae
Through a Dorsal Incision

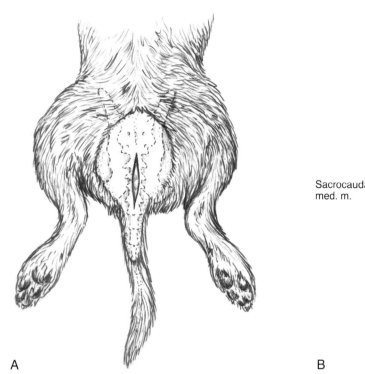

A

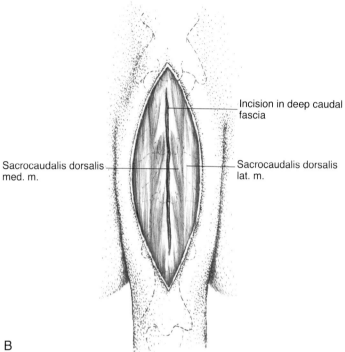

Incision in deep caudal
fascia

Sacrocaudalis dorsalis
med. m.

Sacrocaudalis dorsalis
lat. m.

B

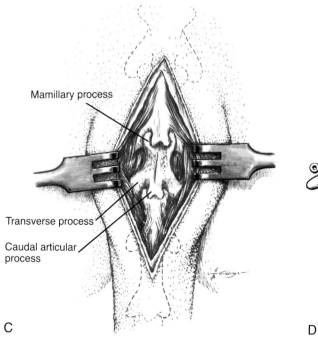

Mamillary process

Transverse process

Caudal articular
process

C

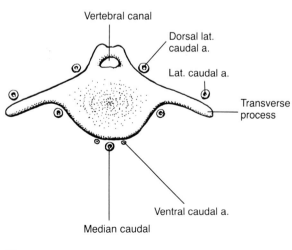

Vertebral canal

Dorsal lat.
caudal a.

Lat. caudal a.

Transverse
process

Ventral caudal a.

Median caudal

D

The Scapula and Shoulder Joint

- Approach to the Body, Spine, and Acromion Process of the Scapula

- Approach to the Craniolateral Region of the Shoulder Joint

- Approach to the Craniolateral Region of the Shoulder Joint by Tenotomy of the Infraspinatus Muscle

- Approach to the Caudolateral Region of the Shoulder Joint

- Approach to the Caudal Region of the Shoulder Joint

- Approach to the Craniomedial Region of the Shoulder Joint

- Approach to the Cranial Region of the Shoulder Joint

Approach to the Body, Spine, and Acromion Process of the Scapula

Based on a Procedure of Alexander[1]

INDICATION

Open reduction of fractures of the scapula.

ALTERNATIVE/COMBINATION APPROACHES

Plates 23 and 28

DESCRIPTION OF THE PROCEDURE

A. The skin and subcutaneous fascial incision is made directly on the spine of the scapula. The skin and fascia are retracted following the undermining of the edges of the incision. The length of the incision is adjusted to fit the area of interest in the exposure.

B. An incision is now made in the deep fascia along the spine of the scapula and is deepened to free the origin of the scapular part of the deltoideus and the insertions of the omotransversarius and trapezius muscles. These muscles are freed and retracted sufficiently to expose the spine and spinatus muscles.

C. The infraspinatus and supraspinatus muscles are elevated from the spine of the scapula. The bellies of the muscles can then be bluntly undermined and retracted from the body of the scapula. Near the acromion, an incision can be made a short distance into the septum between the acromial and scapular parts of the deltoideus to allow retraction of the scapular part.

CLOSURE

A single row of sutures will suffice to close all the incised deep structures. The suture line runs directly along the spine and includes the deep fascia and the omotransversarius, trapezius, and deltoideus muscles. Subcutaneous tissues and skin are closed in separate layers.

COMMENTS

Elevation of the infraspinatus muscle from the scapular spine is complicated by the presence of the metacromion in the *cat*. This caudally projecting protuberance, located on the spine 1 to 2 cm proximal to the acromion, overhangs the infraspinatus slightly, but it does not actually alter the procedure.

Plate 22
Approach to the Body, Spine, and Acromion Process of the Scapula

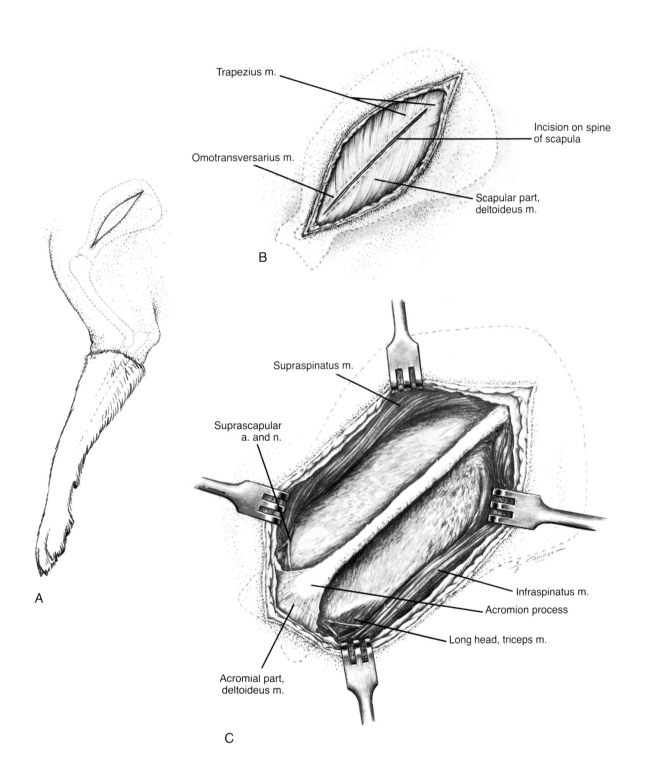

Trapezius m.

Incision on spine of scapula

Omotransversarius m.

Scapular part, deltoideus m.

B

Supraspinatus m.

Suprascapular a. and n.

Infraspinatus m.

Acromion process

Long head, triceps m.

Acromial part, deltoideus m.

A

C

Approach to the Craniolateral Region of the Shoulder Joint

INDICATIONS

1. Open reduction of fractures of the neck and glenoid cavity of the scapula.
2. Open reduction of luxations of the shoulder joint.
3. Osteochondroplasty for osteochondritis of the humeral head.
4. Open reduction of fractures of the humeral head.

ALTERNATIVE/COMBINATION APPROACHES

Plates 22 and 28

DESCRIPTION OF THE PROCEDURE

A. The curved incision begins at the middle of the scapula and follows the spine distally, crossing the joint and continuing over the lateral surface of the humerus to the midpoint of the shaft. The skin margins are undermined and retracted after the subcutaneous fascia and fat are incised in the same line as the skin incision.

B. An incision is made in the deep fascia, starting distally at the omobrachial vein and centered over the belly of the acromial part of the deltoideus. It continues proximally toward the acromial process, passing through the craniodistal insertion of the omotransversarius muscle, and onto the spine of the scapula. The scapular incision encompasses the distal one third of the spine and is deepened both dorsal and ventral to the spine to include the insertions of the omotransversarius and trapezius and the origin of the scapular part of the deltoideus muscle. Take care not to incise the underlying spinatus muscles.

C. The omotransversarius and trapezius are retracted craniodorsad. An incision is made between the two parts of the deltoideus (shown in illustration A of the plate) and is developed bluntly to allow freeing of the scapular part of the deltoideus and its caudoventral retraction. Use care during this dissection to preserve as many as possible of the muscular branches of the axillary nerve that will be found in this area. The area of the acromion is cleared of adherent tissue to allow an osteotomy.

Plate 23

Approach to the Craniolateral Region of the Shoulder Joint

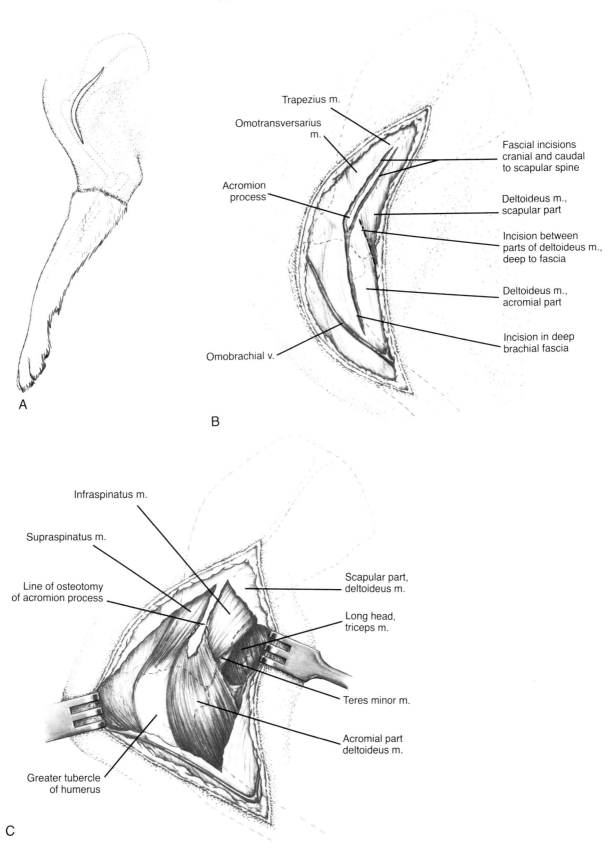

Trapezius m.

Omotransversarius m.

Acromion process

Omobrachial v.

Fascial incisions cranial and caudal to scapular spine

Deltoideus m., scapular part

Incision between parts of deltoideus m., deep to fascia

Deltoideus m., acromial part

Incision in deep brachial fascia

A

B

Infraspinatus m.

Supraspinatus m.

Line of osteotomy of acromion process

Scapular part, deltoideus m.

Long head, triceps m.

Teres minor m.

Acromial part deltoideus m.

Greater tubercle of humerus

C

Approach to the Craniolateral Region of the Shoulder Joint *continued*

DESCRIPTION OF THE PROCEDURE *continued*

D. The acromion is osteotomized to include all the origin of the acromial part of the deltoideus. Either an osteotome or a bone-cutting forceps can be used for the cut; in either case, care must be used to protect the underlying suprascapular nerve. Some surgeons prefer and some circumstances dictate tenotomy of the origin of the deltoideus near the acromion (see "Comments" below). Protect the branches of the axillary nerve entering the deep surface of the muscle as it is retracted distally.

E. The supraspinatus and infraspinatus muscles are bluntly elevated from the spine and body of the scapula sufficiently to allow their retraction as shown. Note the position of the suprascapular nerve and avoid this structure during the elevation and retraction of the infraspinatus.

  Exposure of the joint requires tenotomy of the infraspinatus muscle. This cut is made near the muscle's insertion on the humerus, with enough stump being left to receive one or two sutures. In some cases it may be necessary to treat the teres minor muscle in a like manner, thus allowing greater exposure of the ventrolateral aspect of the joint capsule.

CLOSURE

A modified Bunnell-Mayer or locking-loop suture (Fig. 21A, C), reinforced with one or two mattress sutures, is used to join the severed infraspinatus. The acromion is attached to the spine by two 20- to 22-gauge monofilament stainless steel sutures placed through holes drilled in the bones. Several sutures are placed between the two parts of the deltoideus muscle. A single tier of sutures may be used to close the remaining muscles and deep fascia. Starting at the proximal end of the incision the stitch engages the deep fascia, the trapezius, the scapular part of the deltoideus, and the deep fascia. This pattern is continued distally, with the omotransversarius replacing the trapezius as the acromion is approached. Distal to the acromion, the deep fascia alone is closed.

COMMENTS

Elevation of the infraspinatus muscle from the scapular spine is complicated by the presence of the metacromion in the *cat*. This caudally projecting protuberance, located 1 to 2 cm proximal to the acromion, overhangs the infraspinatus slightly, but it does not actually alter the procedure.

In very young animals the acromion may not yet be ossified. In these cases, a tenotomy of the acromial part of the deltoideus is done close to the acromion. This is also probably more satisfactory in small dogs and cats. Holes drilled in the acromion allow for reattachment of the tendon.

The exposure provided here is generally much greater than is needed for osteochondritis dissecans surgery. It is advised for this only when the surgeon has no assistant to retract and position the limb, as is needed in the other recommended approaches.

Plate 23

Approach to the Craniolateral Region
of the Shoulder Joint *continued*

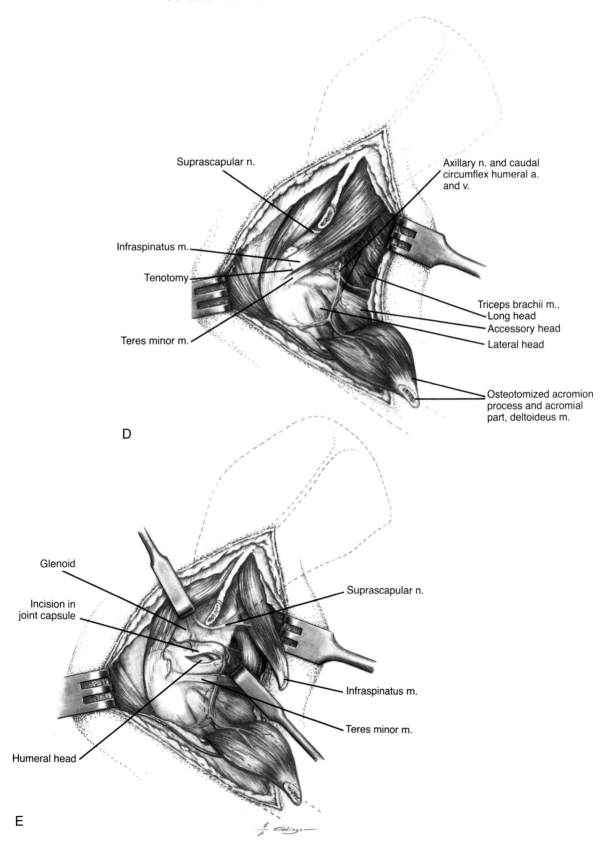

Suprascapular n.

Axillary n. and caudal circumflex humeral a. and v.

Infraspinatus m.

Tenotomy

Teres minor m.

Triceps brachii m., Long head
Accessory head
Lateral head

Osteotomized acromion process and acromial part, deltoideus m.

D

Glenoid

Incision in joint capsule

Suprascapular n.

Infraspinatus m.

Teres minor m.

Humeral head

E

Approach to the Craniolateral Region of the Shoulder Joint by Tenotomy of the Infraspinatus Muscle

Based on a Procedure of Hohn[16]

INDICATIONS

1. Osteochondroplasty of humeral head for osteochondritis dissecans.
2. Tenotomy for contracture of the infraspinatus muscle.

ALTERNATIVE/COMBINATION APPROACHES

Plates 23 and 25

DESCRIPTION OF THE PROCEDURE

A. A curved incision begins at the distal one third of the scapular spine and follows the spine distally, crossing the joint and continuing over the craniolateral surface of the humerus to the midshaft region. Skin margins are undermined and retracted after the subcutaneous fat and fascia are incised in the same line as the skin.

B. Deep fascia is incised, beginning at the acromion and continuing distally over the cranial border of the acromial part of the deltoideus. This incision is continued to the insertion of the acromial part of the deltoideus on the humerus.

C. The belly of the acromial part of the deltoideus is retracted to allow tenotomy of the infraspinatus tendon 5 mm from its humeral insertion. Elevation of a portion of the insertion of the deltoideus may be necessary to obtain adequate retraction of this muscle.

Plate 24

Approach to the Craniolateral Region of the Shoulder Joint by Tenotomy of the Infraspinatus Muscle

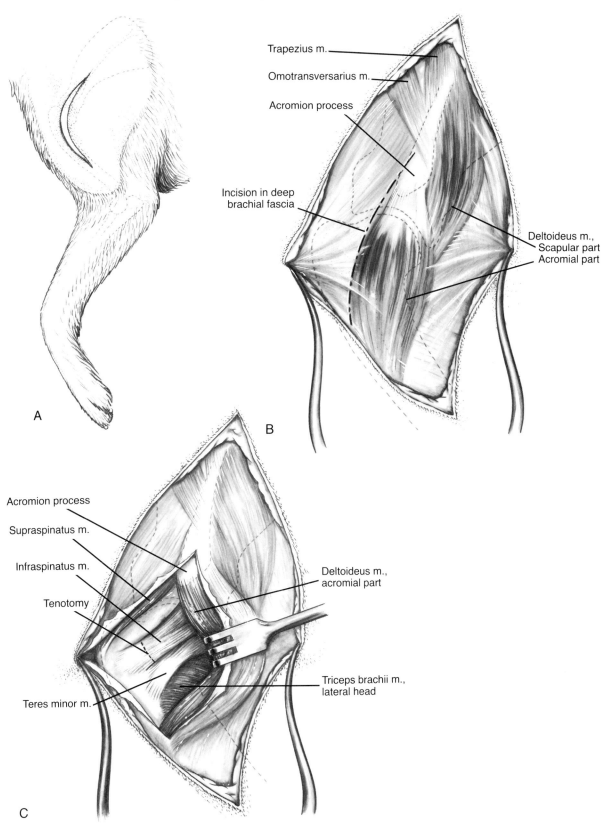

Trapezius m.

Omotransversarius m.

Acromion process

Incision in deep brachial fascia

Deltoideus m., Scapular part Acromial part

A

B

Acromion process

Supraspinatus m.

Infraspinatus m.

Tenotomy

Teres minor m.

Deltoideus m., acromial part

Triceps brachii m., lateral head

C

Approach to the Craniolateral Region of the Shoulder Joint by Tenotomy of the Infraspinatus Muscle *continued*

DESCRIPTION OF THE PROCEDURE *continued*

D. Retraction of the infraspinatus tendon and acromial part of the deltoideus will allow incision of the joint capsule midway between the glenoid rim and the humeral head. Additional exposure can be obtained by tenotomy of the tendon of the teres minor muscle.

E. After retraction of the joint capsule, the humerus is strongly rotated internally to increase exposure of the caudal portion of the head. The humeral head can be partially luxated in the lateral direction for best exposure of a large lesion.

CLOSURE

The joint capsule is closed with interrupted absorbable sutures of 3/0 size. The tendon of the infraspinatus is reattached with a modified Bunnell-Mayer suture (Figure 21A) and reinforced with one or two mattress sutures, nonabsorbable material of 0 or 2/0 size being used. The deep fascial incision, subcutaneous fat and fascia, and skin are closed in separate layers.

COMMENTS

This approach gives better exposure to the humeral head than the caudolateral approach to the shoulder (Plate 25), but poorer access to the caudal compartment of the joint for removal of joint mice.

Plate 24

Approach to the Craniolateral Region of the Shoulder Joint by Tenotomy of the Infraspinatus Muscle *continued*

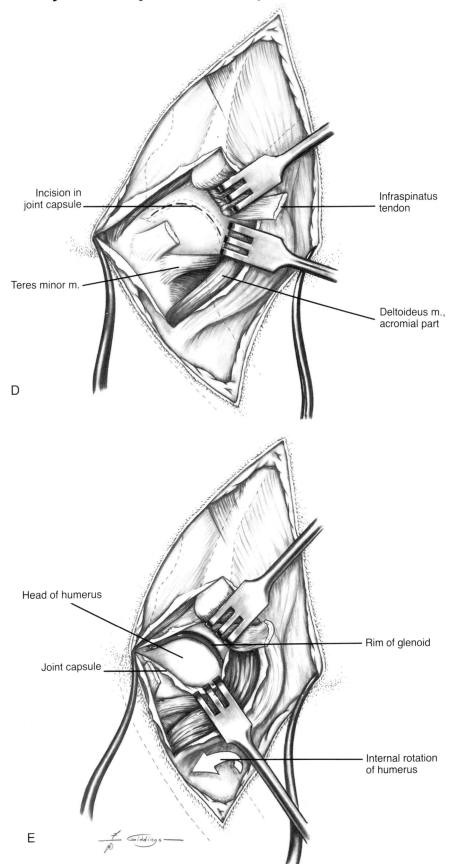

Incision in joint capsule

Infraspinatus tendon

Teres minor m.

Deltoideus m., acromial part

D

Head of humerus

Rim of glenoid

Joint capsule

Internal rotation of humerus

E

Giddings

Approach to the Caudolateral Region of the Shoulder Joint

INDICATIONS

1. Osteochondroplasty of humeral head for osteochondritis dissecans.
2. Open reduction of caudoventral luxations of the shoulder.
3. Open reduction of fractures of the ventral portion of the glenoid cavity.

ALTERNATIVE/COMBINATION APPROACHES

Plates 23, 24, and 26

DESCRIPTION OF THE PROCEDURE

A. A curved incision begins at the middle of the scapula and follows the spine distally, crossing the joint and continuing over the lateral surface of the humerus to the midpoint of the shaft. Skin margins are undermined and retracted after subcutaneous fascia and fat are incised in the same line as the skin incision.

B. Deep fascia is incised over the ventral border of the distal scapular spine to free the origin of the scapular part of the deltoideus muscle. This fascial incision is continued distally over the acromial part of the deltoideus to the omobrachial vein. The incised fascia is elevated and retracted cranially and caudally from the underlying deltoideus muscle.

C. An incision is made on the ventral border of the spine of the scapula and continued distally between the spinous and acromial parts of the deltoideus muscle.

Plate 25

Approach to the Caudolateral Region of the Shoulder Joint

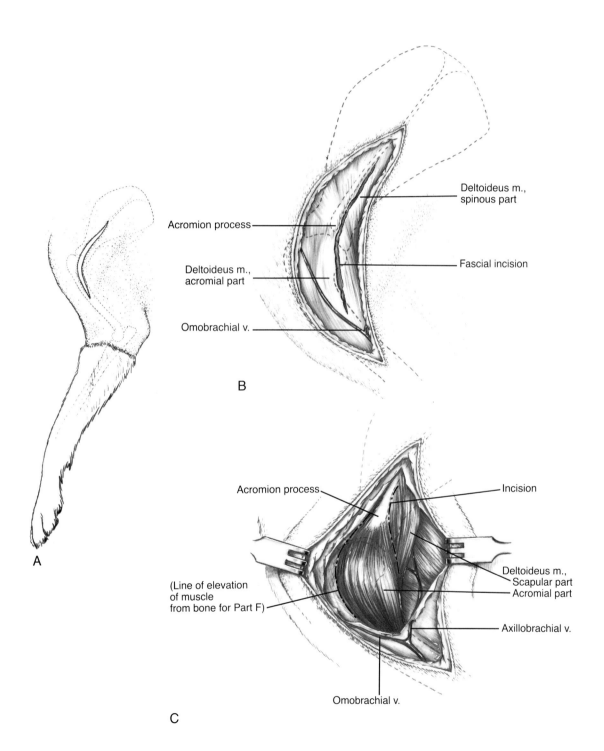

Deltoideus m., spinous part

Acromion process

Deltoideus m., acromial part

Fascial incision

Omobrachial v.

B

A

Acromion process

Incision

(Line of elevation of muscle from bone for Part F)

Deltoideus m., Scapular part
Acromial part

Axillobrachial v.

Omobrachial v.

C

Approach to the Caudolateral Region of the Shoulder Joint *continued*

DESCRIPTION OF THE PROCEDURE *continued*

D. The division between the two parts of deltoideus muscle is developed by blunt dissection to allow freeing of the spinous part of the muscle and its caudal retraction with the deep fascia. A muscular branch of the axillary nerve is found between the two parts of the deltoideus. It is usually possible to preserve this structure.

N.B. There are two possible ways to proceed from this point. Part E illustrates the simpler method, but it may not provide sufficient exposure in some animals. Continuing as in Parts F and G will give additional exposure.

E. Strong dorsocranial retraction of the teres minor muscle will expose the joint capsule. An incision is made parallel and close to the rim of the glenoid cavity. Care is taken to protect the subscapular vessels and axillary nerve lying between the joint capsule and the long head of the triceps muscle. Internal rotation and adduction of the humerus provides maximal exposure of the humeral head.

Plate 25

Approach to the Caudolateral Region of the Shoulder Joint *continued*

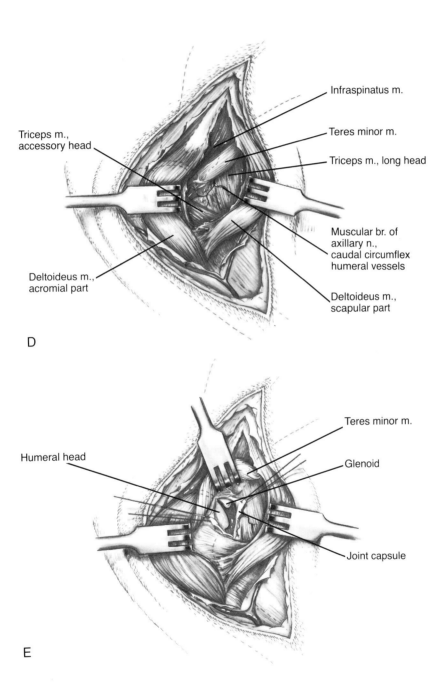

D

Triceps m., accessory head

Deltoideus m., acromial part

Infraspinatus m.

Teres minor m.

Triceps m., long head

Muscular br. of axillary n., caudal circumflex humeral vessels

Deltoideus m., scapular part

E

Humeral head

Teres minor m.

Glenoid

Joint capsule

Approach to the Caudolateral Region of the Shoulder Joint *continued*

DESCRIPTION OF THE PROCEDURE *continued*

F. The belly of the acromial part of the deltoideus is undermined and elevated from the underlying humerus (see incision in illustration C). The deltoideus is then retracted caudally to expose the tendons of insertion of the infraspinatus and teres minor muscles on the greater tubercle of the humerus. Fascia overlying the tendon of the teres minor is incised to allow tenotomy about 5 mm from its insertion. It is helpful to place a modified mattress or locking-loop suture in the tendon before its transection. Nonabsorbable suture material is used.

G. The tendon suture is passed caudally under the acromial part of the deltoideus, and the two bellies of this muscle are retracted. The tendon suture in the teres minor is used to apply traction as the muscle is dissected free from the underlying joint capsule. The infraspinatus is retracted dorsally and the joint capsule is incised parallel to the rim of the glenoid. As this incision is carried caudally to the flexor surface of the joint, care must be taken to preserve the subscapular artery and axillary nerve that lie very close to the joint. Internal rotation of the humerus will provide maximum exposure of the caudal surface of the humeral head.

CLOSURE

The joint capsule is closed with interrupted sutures of 3/0 absorbable material. If the teres minor tendon was cut, the preplaced tendon suture is placed through the tendon insertion and tied. External rotation of the humerus will facilitate tying this suture. Additional small mattress sutures are used in the tendon if necessary to gain adequate closure. The intermuscular septum between the two parts of the deltoideus is next sutured with any suture material of choice and the cranial border of the acromial part of the deltoideus is reattached to the fascia on the proximal portion of the humeral shaft. The next step is to suture the fascial origin of the spinous part of the deltoideus to the spine of the scapula. This suture line is continued distally to close the fascia overlying the acromial part of the deltoideus. Subcutaneous closure is made with care, due to a tendency for subcutaneous seroma formation.

COMMENTS

This approach gives good exposure for removal of joint mice in the caudal compartment of the shoulder joint, although exposure of the humeral head lesion of osteochondritis is more limited than in the craniolateral approaches (Plates 23 and 24).

Plate 25

Approach to the Caudolateral Region
of the Shoulder Joint *continued*

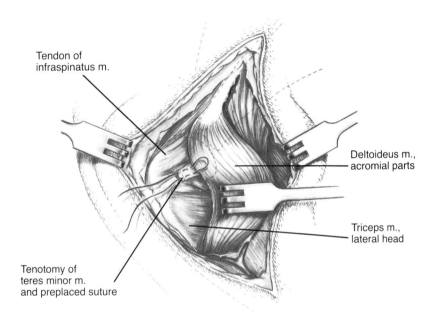

Tendon of
infraspinatus m.

Deltoideus m.,
acromial parts

Triceps m.,
lateral head

Tenotomy of
teres minor m.
and preplaced suture

F

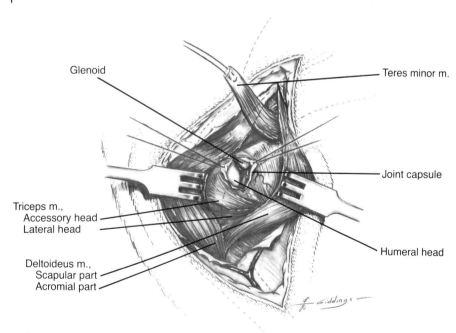

Glenoid

Teres minor m.

Joint capsule

Triceps m.,
Accessory head
Lateral head

Deltoideus m.,
Scapular part
Acromial part

Humeral head

G

Approach to the Caudal Region of the Shoulder Joint

Based on a Procedure of Gahring [12]

INDICATION

Osteochondroplasty for osteochondritis dissecans of the humeral head.

ALTERNATIVE/COMBINATION APPROACHES

Plates 23, 24, and 25

DESCRIPTION OF THE PROCEDURE

A. The skin incision extends from the middle of the scapular spine to the midshaft of the humerus.

B. Subcutaneous fat and deep fascia of the shoulder are incised and elevated to reveal the scapular part of the deltoideus muscle and the lateral and long heads of the triceps brachii muscle. An incision is made in the intermuscular septum between the caudal border of the deltoideus and the long head of the triceps, and continued distally over the lateral head of the triceps.

C. Blunt dissection under the deltoideus and strong elevation of that muscle will reveal the caudal circumflex artery and vein and a muscular branch of the axillary nerve. The teres minor muscle and the joint capsule lie directly under these structures.

Plate 26

Approach to the Caudal Region of the Shoulder Joint

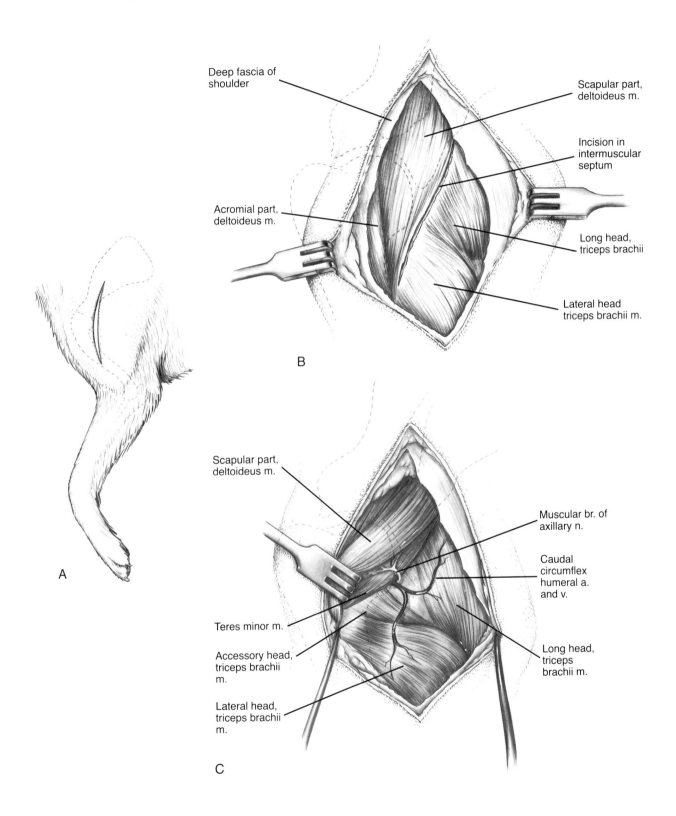

Deep fascia of shoulder

Scapular part, deltoideus m.

Incision in intermuscular septum

Acromial part, deltoideus m.

Long head, triceps brachii

Lateral head triceps brachii m.

B

Scapular part, deltoideus m.

Muscular br. of axillary n.

Caudal circumflex humeral a. and v.

Teres minor m.

Accessory head, triceps brachii m.

Long head, triceps brachii m.

Lateral head, triceps brachii m.

A

C

Approach to the Caudal Region of the Shoulder Joint *continued*

DESCRIPTION OF THE PROCEDURE *continued*

D. Craniodorsal retraction of the teres minor will expose the axillary nerve.

E. The axillary nerve and accompanying vessels are elevated and retracted with a rubber Penrose drain or umbilical tape. Palpation will identify the inferior rim of the glenoid cavity and the caudal aspect of the humeral head. The joint capsule is incised 5 mm from and parallel to the rim of the glenoid cavity.

Plate 26

Approach to the Caudal Region of the Shoulder Joint *continued*

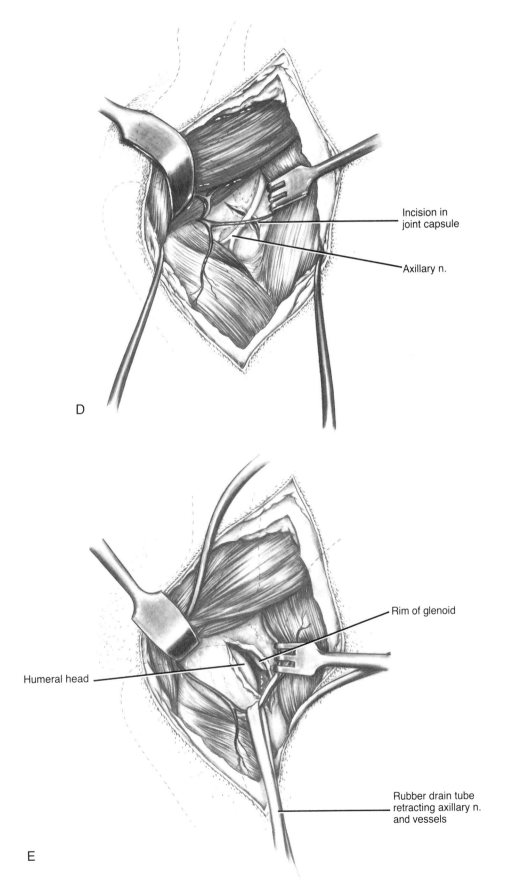

Incision in
joint capsule

Axillary n.

D

Rim of glenoid

Humeral head

Rubber drain tube
retracting axillary n.
and vessels

E

Approach to the Caudal Region of the Shoulder Joint *continued*

DESCRIPTION OF THE PROCEDURE *continued*

F. Retraction of the joint capsule gives good exposure of the caudal cul-de-sac of the joint. Strong internal rotation of the limb, combined with varying degrees of flexion and extension of the shoulder, will provide exposure of the osteochondritis lesion.

CLOSURE

The joint capsule is closed with interrupted sutures of 3/0 absorbable material. The intermuscular septum between the deltoideus and triceps muscles is closed, followed by closure of the deep fascial layer, subcutaneous tissues, and skin.

COMMENTS

This approach gives good exposure of the humeral head and the caudal cul-de-sac, where loose cartilage fragments gravitate. It has the advantage of not involving any tenotomies.

Plate 26

Approach to the Caudal Region of the Shoulder Joint *continued*

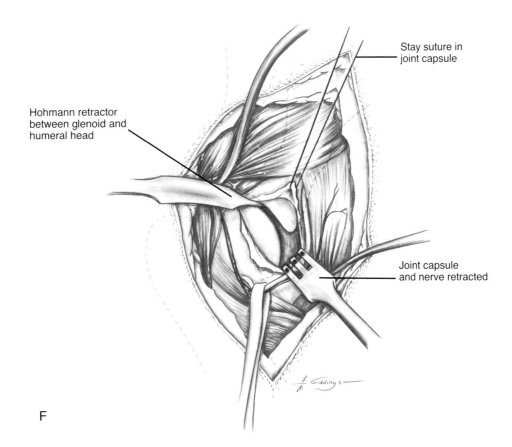

Stay suture in
joint capsule

Hohmann retractor
between glenoid and
humeral head

Joint capsule
and nerve retracted

F

Approach to the Craniomedial Region of the Shoulder Joint

Based on a Procedure of Hohn et al.[19]

INDICATIONS

1. Open reduction of medial shoulder luxations.
2. Open reduction of fractures of the neck and glenoid cavity of the scapula.
3. Open reduction of fractures of the lesser tubercle of the humerus.

ALTERNATIVE/COMBINATION APPROACHES

Plates 23 and 27

DESCRIPTION OF THE PROCEDURE

A. The skin incision starts medial to and slightly caudal to the acromion of the scapula. It continues distally, medial to the midline of the humerus, and ends at the midshaft of this bone. The dog is in dorsal recumbency.

B. After incision and retraction of the subcutaneous tissues with the skin, the brachiocephalicus muscle is identified. This muscle is retracted medially, following a fascial incision along its lateral border for the entire length of the exposure. The omobrachial vein is ligated to allow this incision.

C. The limb is externally rotated and the insertion of the superficial pectoral muscle is freed from the humerus from its proximal border distally to the cephalic vein, which crosses the muscle. This muscle will not be reattached at its insertion, so it can be cut very close to the bone.

Plate 27

Approach to the Craniomedial Region of the Shoulder Joint

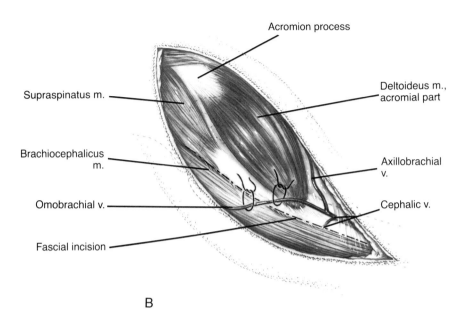

Acromion process

Supraspinatus m.

Deltoideus m., acromial part

Brachiocephalicus m.

Axillobrachial v.

Omobrachial v.

Cephalic v.

Fascial incision

B

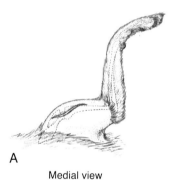

A

Medial view

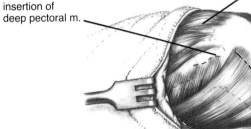
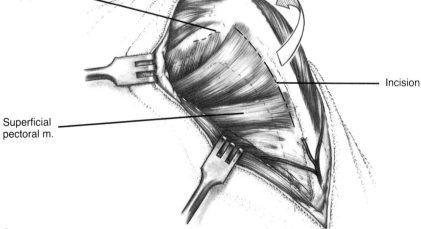

Supraspinatus m.

Incision in insertion of deep pectoral m.

Incision

Superficial pectoral m.

C

Approach to the Craniomedial Region of the Shoulder Joint *continued*

DESCRIPTION OF THE PROCEDURE *continued*

D. The deep pectoral is similarly incised to free its entire insertion. After separating the fascial attachments between the supraspinatus and the deep pectoral, both pectoral muscles are retracted medially. When separating the deep pectoral from the supraspinatus muscle, be aware of the position of the suprascapular nerve (see illustration A, Plate 28). The tendon of the coracobrachialis muscle is incised near its insertion. This exposes the tendon of insertion of the subscapularis muscle on the lesser tubercle of the humerus.

E. The tendinous insertion of the subscapularis muscle on the lesser tubercle of the humerus is cut close to the bone, but enough tendon is left on the bone to allow suturing. The joint capsule is incised parallel to the medial rim of the glenoid cavity. Retraction of the belly of the subscapularis muscle exposes the medial joint capsule, which is incised as needed to gain access to the interior of the joint.

CLOSURE

The joint capsule is sutured with 2/0 to 3/0 interrupted absorbable sutures. Mattress sutures of 0 to 2/0 nonabsorbable material are used to reattach the tendon of the subscapularis muscle. Both pectoral muscles are advanced cranially to attach to deltoideus and deep brachial fascia. The brachiocephalicus muscle is sutured to brachial fascia, and subcutaneous tissues are closed in layers.

Plate 27

Approach to the Craniomedial Region
of the Shoulder Joint *continued*

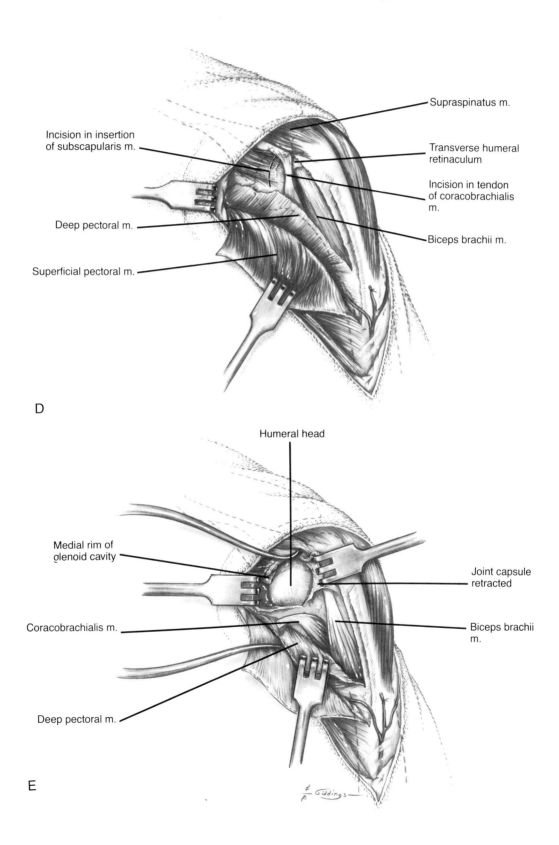

Incision in insertion
of subscapularis m.

Deep pectoral m.

Superficial pectoral m.

Supraspinatus m.

Transverse humeral
retinaculum

Incision in tendon
of coracobrachialis
m.

Biceps brachii m.

D

Humeral head

Medial rim of
glenoid cavity

Coracobrachialis m.

Deep pectoral m.

Joint capsule
retracted

Biceps brachii
m.

E

Approach to the Cranial Region of the Shoulder Joint

Based on a Procedure of De Angelis and Schwartz [9]

INDICATIONS

1. Open reduction of cranial luxations of the shoulder.
2. Open reduction of fractures of the neck and glenoid of the scapula (see "Comments" below).
3. Open reduction of fractures of the head of the humerus.

ALTERNATIVE/COMBINATION APPROACHES

Plates 23 and 27

EXPLANATORY NOTE

The procedure is initiated as shown in Parts A through D of Plate 27, Approach to the Craniomedial Region of the Shoulder Joint.

DESCRIPTION OF THE PROCEDURE

A, B. Following elevation and retraction of the superficial and deep pectoral muscles, the fascial attachments between the deep pectoral and supraspinatus muscles are divided sufficiently to allow retraction of the supraspinatus. An osteotome is used to osteotomize the greater tubercle containing the tendinous insertion of the supraspinatus muscle. Note that the cut is made at two different angles, in order to better resist the shearing forces of muscle pull after reattachment. Care must be taken to not cut the tendinous insertion of the infraspinatus muscle and to protect the tendon of the biceps muscle during the osteotomy.

Plate 28

Approach to the Cranial Region of the Shoulder Joint

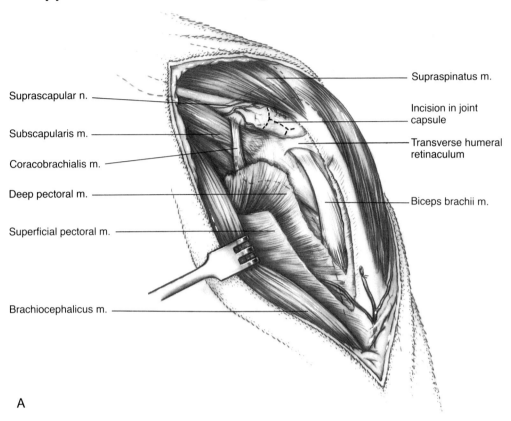

Suprascapular n.

Subscapularis m.

Coracobrachialis m.

Deep pectoral m.

Superficial pectoral m.

Brachiocephalicus m.

Supraspinatus m.

Incision in joint capsule

Transverse humeral retinaculum

Biceps brachii m.

A

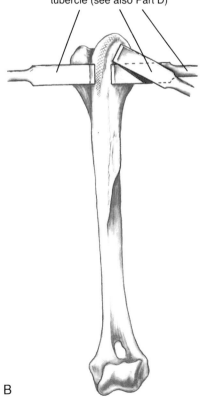

Position of osteotome for osteotomy of the greater tubercle (see also Part D)

B

Approach to the Cranial Region of the Shoulder Joint *continued*

DESCRIPTION OF THE PROCEDURE *continued*

C. The supraspinatus muscle can now be reflected proximally and dorsally after dissecting it free of the joint capsule. Continued elevation of the muscle from the scapula will expose the scapular neck and glenoid. Identify and protect the suprascapular nerve (also see Part E, Plate 23).

CLOSURE

The greater tubercle is reattached with two lag screws or two Kirschner wires of 0.045- to 0.062-inch diameter as shown in illustration D. The superficial and deep pectoral muscles are sutured to the fascia of the deltoideus muscle. The remaining fascial layers, subcutaneous tissues, and skin are closed separately.

COMMENTS

For total exposure of the scapular neck and most of the glenoid cavity, this approach is combined with the Approach to the Craniolateral Region of the Shoulder Joint (Plate 23).

Plate 28

Approach to the Cranial Region of the Shoulder Joint *continued*

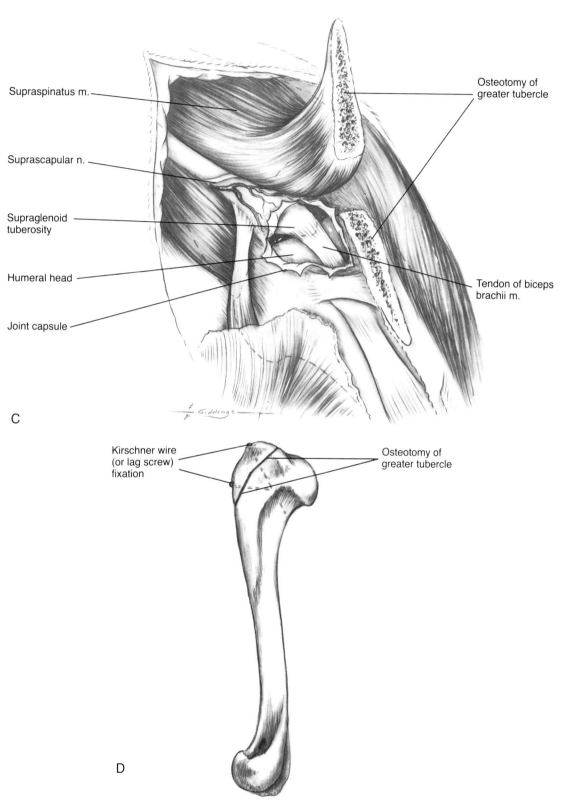

Supraspinatus m.

Suprascapular n.

Supraglenoid tuberosity

Humeral head

Joint capsule

Osteotomy of greater tubercle

Tendon of biceps brachii m.

C

Kirschner wire (or lag screw) fixation

Osteotomy of greater tubercle

D

The Thoracic Limb

- Approach to the Proximal Shaft of the Humerus

- Approach to the Shaft of the Humerus Through a Craniolateral Incision

- Approach to the Shaft of the Humerus Through a Medial Incision

- Approach to the Distal Shaft of the Humerus Through a Craniolateral Incision

- Approach to the Distal Shaft and Supracondylar Region of the Humerus Through a Medial Incision

- Approach to the Lateral Aspect of the Humeral Condyle and Epicondyle

- Approach to the Lateral Humeroulnar Part of the Elbow Joint

- Approach to the Supracondylar Region of the Humerus and the Caudal Humeroulnar Part of the Elbow Joint

- Approach to the Humeroulnar Part of the Elbow Joint by Osteotomy of the Tuber Olecrani

- Approach to the Elbow Joint by Osteotomy of the Proximal Ulnar Diaphysis

- Approach to the Head of the Radius and Lateral Parts of the Elbow Joint

- Approach to the Head of the Radius and Humeroradial Part of the Elbow Joint by Osteotomy of the Lateral Humeral Epicondyle

- Approach to the Medial Humeral Epicondyle

- Approach to the Medial Aspect of the Humeral Condyle and the Medial Coronoid Process of the Ulna by an Intermuscular Incision

- Approach to the Medial Aspect of the Humeral Condyle and the Medial Coronoid Process of the Ulna by Osteotomy of the Medial Humeral Epicondyle

- Approach to the Proximal Shaft and Trochlear Notch of the Ulna

- Approach to the Tuber Olecrani

- Approach to the Distal Shaft and Styloid Process of the Ulna

- Approach to the Head and Proximal Metaphysis of the Radius

- Approach to the Shaft of the Radius Through a Medial Incision

- Approach to the Shaft of the Radius Through a Lateral Incision

- Approach to the Distal Radius and Carpus Through a Dorsal Incision

- Approach to the Distal Radius and Carpus Through a Palmaromedial Incision

- Approach to the Accessory Carpal Bone and Palmarolateral Carpal Joints

- Approaches to the Metacarpal Bones

- Approach to the Proximal Sesamoid Bones

- Approaches to the Phalanges and Interphalangeal Joints

Approach to the Proximal Shaft of the Humerus

INDICATIONS

Open reduction of fractures of the proximal half of the shaft of the humerus.

ALTERNATIVE/COMBINATION APPROACHES

Plates 30 and 31

DESCRIPTION OF THE PROCEDURE

A. The skin incision is made slightly lateral to the cranial midline of the bone and extends from the greater tubercle of the humerus distally to a point near the midshaft of the bone.

B. Following undermining and retraction of the skin, an incision is made through the deep fascia along the lateral border of the brachiocephalicus muscle. The insertion of the acromial part of the deltoid muscle is also incised.

Plate 29
Approach to the Proximal Shaft of the Humerus

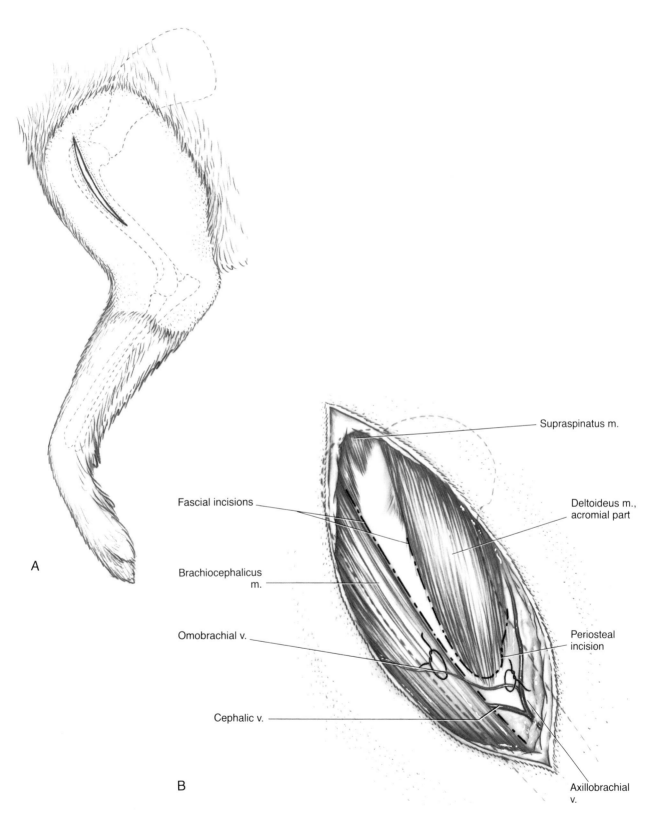

A

B

Supraspinatus m.

Deltoideus m., acromial part

Fascial incisions

Brachiocephalicus m.

Omobrachial v.

Periosteal incision

Cephalic v.

Axillobrachial v.

Approach to the Proximal Shaft of the Humerus *continued*

DESCRIPTION OF THE PROCEDURE *continued*

C. The brachiocephalicus can be retracted cranially following blunt dissection between the muscle and the bone. The deltoideus muscle is retracted caudally to reveal the tendons of insertion of the teres minor and infraspinatus muscles. If more exposure of bone is needed, the insertions of the superficial pectoral muscle and the lateral head of the triceps muscle can be incised.

D. Periosteal elevation of the lateral head of the triceps exposes the lateral and caudal aspects of the shaft. If the craniomedial shaft must be exposed, a portion of the insertion of the deep pectoral muscle can be elevated. This muscle insertion is just medial to that of the superficial pectoral muscle.

CLOSURE

The deep pectoral and triceps muscles are not reattached, because they are only partially elevated and will reattach to the periosteum by fibrosis. The external fascia of the superficial pectoral and deltoideus muscles are sutured to each other over the cranial border of the bone. The deep fascia is reattached to the edge of the brachiocephalicus muscle, followed by closure of the subcutaneous tissues and skin.

Plate 29

Approach to the Proximal Shaft of the Humerus *continued*

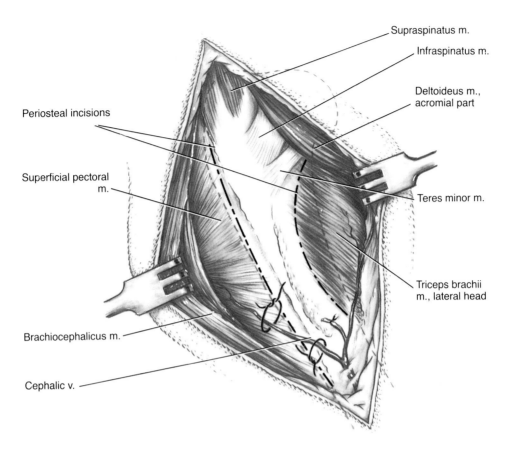

Supraspinatus m.

Infraspinatus m.

Deltoideus m., acromial part

Periosteal incisions

Superficial pectoral m.

Teres minor m.

Triceps brachii m., lateral head

Brachiocephalicus m.

Cephalic v.

C

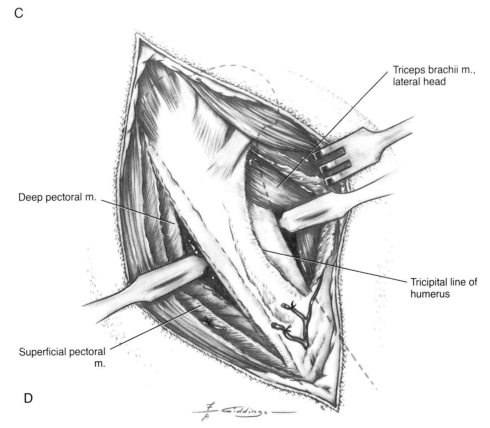

Triceps brachii m., lateral head

Deep pectoral m.

Superficial pectoral m.

Tricipital line of humerus

D

Approach to the Shaft of the Humerus Through a Craniolateral Incision

INDICATION

Internal fixation of shaft fractures.

ALTERNATIVE/COMBINATION APPROACHES

Plates 29, 31, and 32

DESCRIPTION OF THE PROCEDURE

A. The skin incision extends from the greater tubercle of the humerus proximally, to the lateral epicondyle distally, following the craniolateral border of the humerus.

B. Subcutaneous fat and fascia are incised on the same line and mobilized and retracted with the skin. Fat and brachial fascia are incised and dissected away to allow visualization of the cephalic vein. Brachial fascia is incised along the lateral border of the brachiocephalicus muscle and distally over the cephalic vein.

   The cephalic vein is ligated at the distal end of the field and again proximally where it disappears under the edge of the brachiocephalicus muscle. The axillobrachial and omobrachial veins are similarly ligated and the isolated venous segment is removed.

   An incision is made in the craniomedial fascia of the brachialis muscle and in the insertion of the lateral head of the triceps brachii on the humerus.

Plate 30

Approach to the Shaft of the Humerus Through a Craniolateral Incision

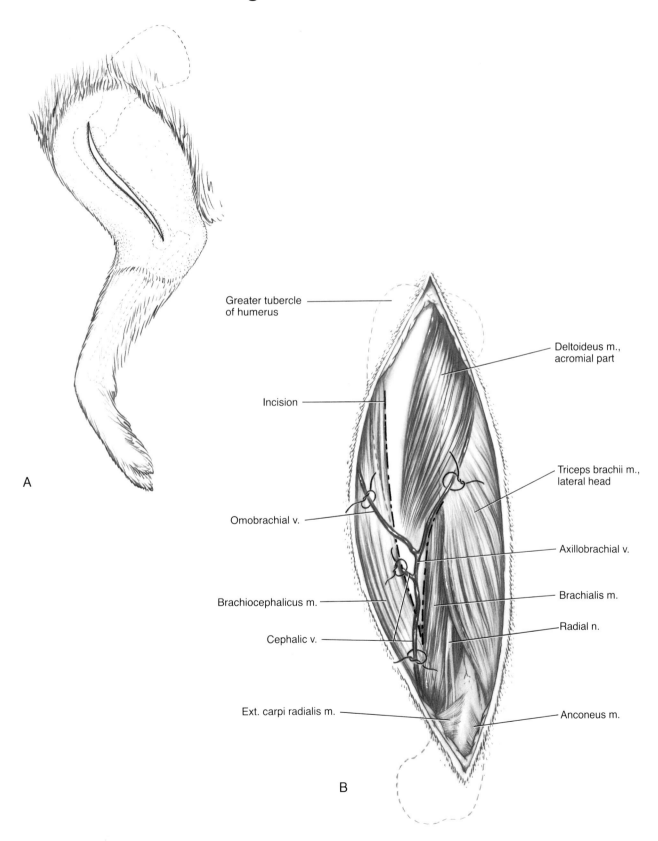

A

Greater tubercle of humerus

Incision

Omobrachial v.

Brachiocephalicus m.

Cephalic v.

Ext. carpi radialis m.

Deltoideus m., acromial part

Triceps brachii m., lateral head

Axillobrachial v.

Brachialis m.

Radial n.

Anconeus m.

B

Approach to the Shaft of the Humerus Through a Craniolateral Incision *continued*

DESCRIPTION OF THE PROCEDURE *continued*

C. An incision is next made in the periosteal insertion of the superficial pectoral and brachiocephalicus muscles on the humeral shaft. The radial nerve should be identified and protected when making these incisions.

D. Hohmann retractors are used to retract the brachialis and triceps muscles caudally and expose the musculospiral groove of the humerus. Cranial retraction will elevate the biceps, superficial pectoral, and brachiocephalicus muscles from the shaft. Again, the radial nerve must be protected during retraction.

CLOSURE

The insertions of the superficial pectoral and brachiocephalicus muscles are sutured to the superficial fascia of the brachialis muscle distally and to the deltoideus muscle proximally. The insertion of the lateral head of the triceps is attached to the brachiocephalicus. Brachial fascia, subcutaneous fat and fascia, and skin are closed in separate layers.

COMMENTS

This approach is used primarily for bone plating or when a long exposure is needed. If additional exposure of the proximal lateral portion of the shaft is required, the deltoid muscle can be elevated subperiostally, as shown in Plate 29. Further exposure of the distal humeral shaft can be obtained by cranial retraction of the brachiocephalicus muscle and radial nerve (see Plate 32, Part E).

Plate 30

Approach to the Shaft of the Humerus
Through a Craniolateral Incision *continued*

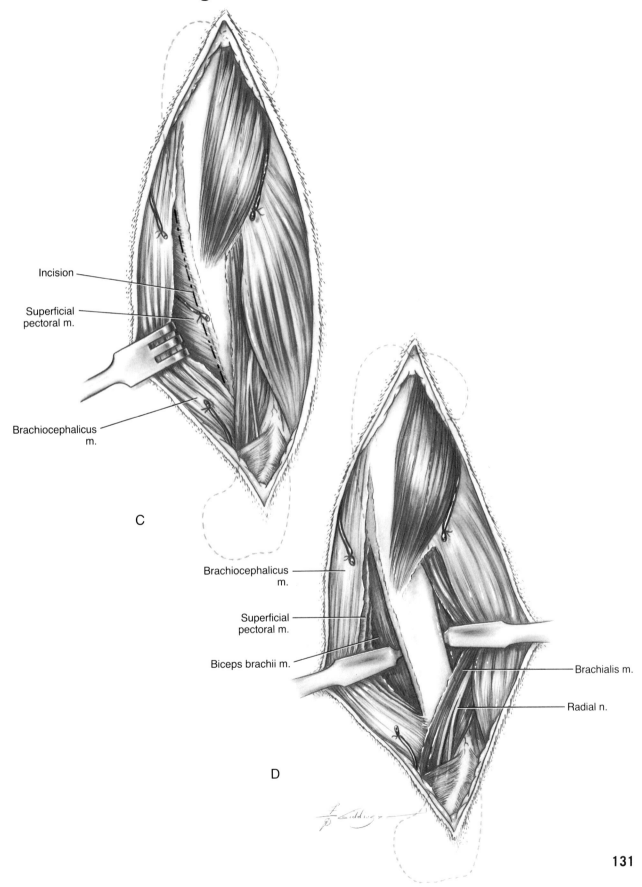

Incision

Superficial
pectoral m.

Brachiocephalicus
m.

C

Brachiocephalicus
m.

Superficial
pectoral m.

Biceps brachii m.

Brachialis m.

Radial n.

D

Approach to the Shaft of the Humerus Through a Medial Incision

Based on a procedure of Montgomery, Milton, and Mann[23]

INDICATION

Open reduction of fractures of the shaft of the humerus.

ALTERNATIVE/COMBINATION APPROACHES

Plates 30, 32, 33, and 34

DESCRIPTION OF THE PROCEDURE

A. The medial skin incision begins proximally at the level of the greater tubercle and extends distally to the medial epicondyle. Subcutaneous fat and fascia are incised on the same line and elevated with the skin.

B. Deep brachial fascia is incised along the caudal border of the brachiocephalicus muscle and along the distal border of the superficial pectoral muscle. The distal part of this incision is made carefully to preserve the underlying neurovascular structures.

Plate 31

Approach to the Shaft of the Humerus
Through a Medial Incision

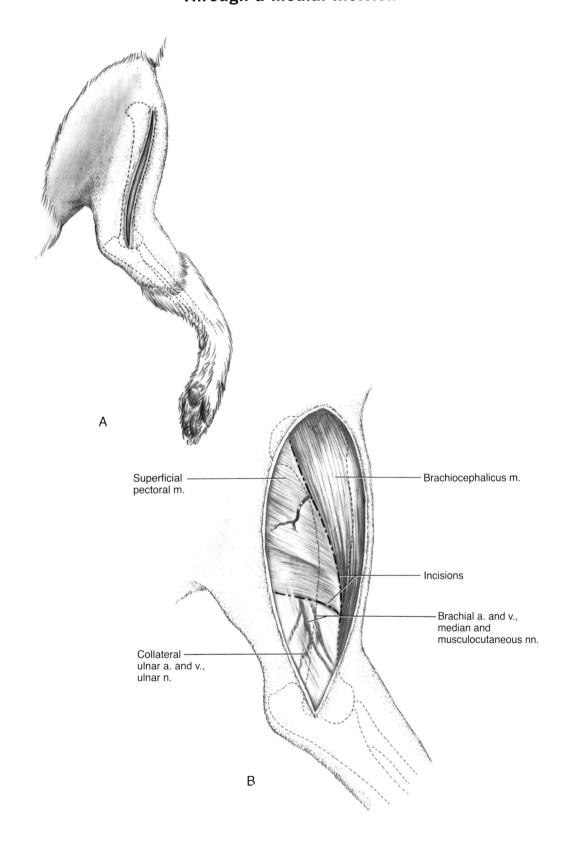

A

Superficial pectoral m.

Brachiocephalicus m.

Incisions

Brachial a. and v., median and musculocutaneous nn.

Collateral ulnar a. and v., ulnar n.

B

Approach to the Shaft of the Humerus Through a Medial Incision *continued*

DESCRIPTION OF THE PROCEDURE *continued*

C. Fascia distal to the superficial pectoral muscle is carefully dissected from the vessels and nerves. The brachiocephalicus muscle is retracted cranially to expose the insertion of the superficial pectoral muscle on the shaft of the humerus. This insertion is incised close to the bone from its distal end proximally to the level of the cephalic vein.

D. The superficial pectoral incision is extended into the muscle parallel to the cephalic vein by blunt dissection between muscle fibers.

Plate 31

Approach to the Shaft of the Humerus
Through a Medial Incision *continued*

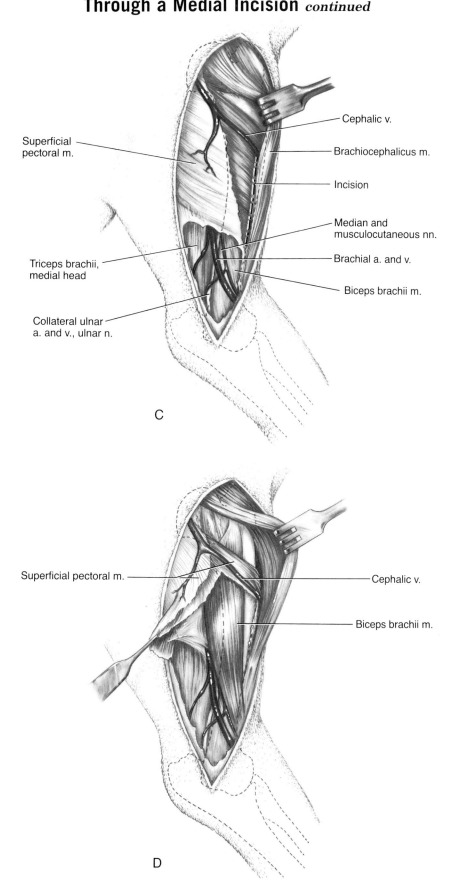

Superficial
pectoral m.

Cephalic v.

Brachiocephalicus m.

Incision

Median and
musculocutaneous nn.

Triceps brachii,
medial head

Brachial a. and v.

Biceps brachii m.

Collateral ulnar
a. and v., ulnar n.

C

Superficial pectoral m.

Cephalic v.

Biceps brachii m.

D

Approach to the Shaft of the Humerus Through a Medial Incision *continued*

DESCRIPTION OF THE PROCEDURE *continued*

E. Exposure of the proximal and midportion of the bone is optimal if the proximal brachiocephalicus muscle is retracted cranially and the biceps brachii muscle is retracted caudally. The remaining attached portion of the superficial pectoral muscle is retracted as necessary, and bone plates are placed under it. If essential, the cephalic vein can be ligated and the entire insertion of the muscle incised.

F. The middle and distal regions of the humerus are best exposed by cranial retraction of the biceps brachii muscle, which requires careful dissection along the caudal border of the muscle to separate it from the neurovascular structures. The proximal and distal branches of the musculocutaneous nerve must be protected where they penetrate the muscle.

CLOSURE

The superficial pectoral muscle is sutured to its insertion or to fascia of the brachialis muscle. The deep fascial incisions are closed, followed by subcutaneous fat and fascia, and skin.

COMMENTS

This approach allows visualization of the entire humerus, which is valuable when applying a bone plate to a highly comminuted fracture. For intramedullary pin fixation, the more limited approaches are usually sufficient.

Plate 31

Approach to the Shaft of the Humerus
Through a Medial Incision *continued*

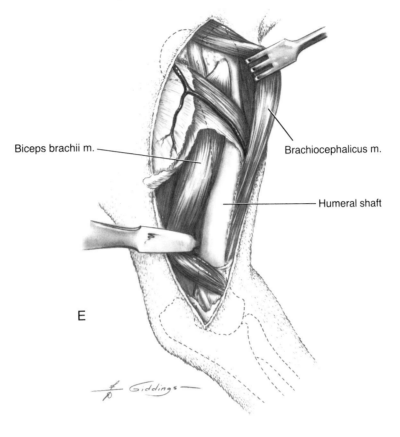

Biceps brachii m.

Brachiocephalicus m.

Humeral shaft

E

Giddings

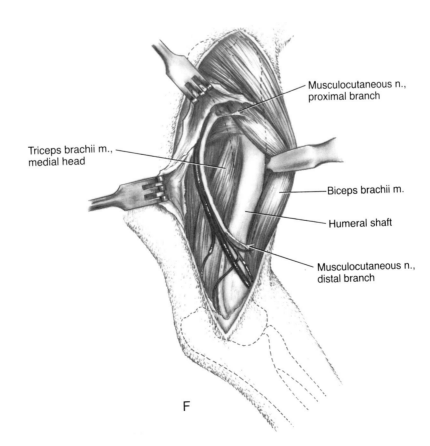

Musculocutaneous n., proximal branch

Triceps brachii m., medial head

Biceps brachii m.

Humeral shaft

Musculocutaneous n., distal branch

F

Approach to the Distal Shaft of the Humerus Through a Craniolateral Incision

Based on a Procedure of Brinker[4]

INDICATION

Open reduction of fractures between the midshaft and the supracondylar area of the humerus.

ALTERNATIVE/COMBINATION APPROACHES

Plates 30, 33, 34, and 36

DESCRIPTION OF THE PROCEDURE

A. The craniolateral border of the humerus is the guide for this incision, which commences at the midshaft and ends at the lateral epicondyle.

B. The skin margins are mobilized and retracted. Subcutaneous fascia and fat are incised in the same line as the skin avoiding the cephalic and axillobrachial veins. The deep fascia of the brachium is incised along the cranial border of the triceps. The incision parallels the cephalic and axillobrachial veins, to allow their mobilization. The radial nerve must be protected when the distal end of this incision is opened.

C. The deep fascia is undermined to allow cranial retraction of the brachiocephalicus muscle and the cephalic vein and exposure of the radial nerve. An incision is made in the periosteal insertion of the superficial pectoral muscle.

Plate 32

Approach to the Distal Shaft of the Humerus Through a Craniolateral Incision

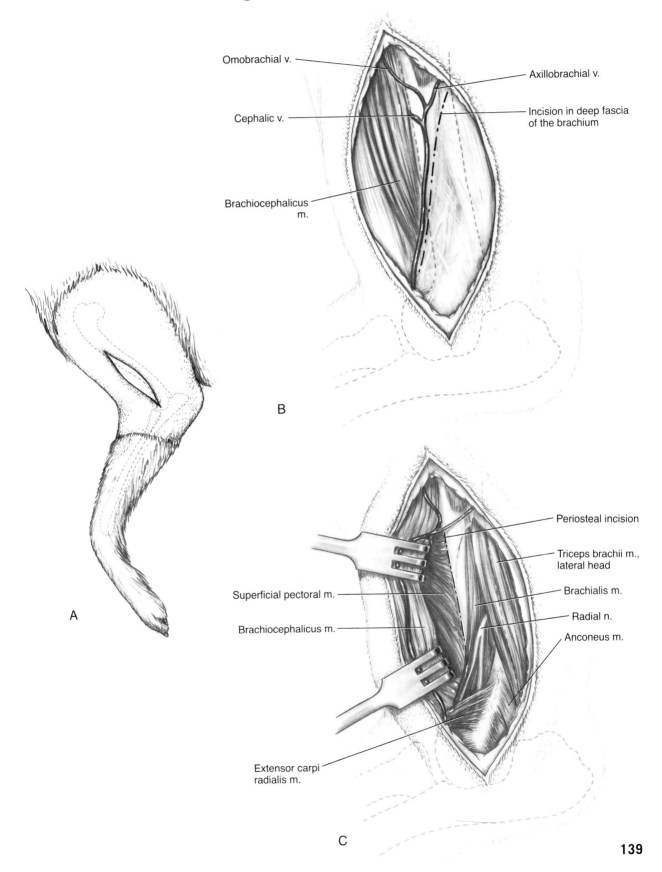

Omobrachial v.

Axillobrachial v.

Cephalic v.

Incision in deep fascia of the brachium

Brachiocephalicus m.

B

Periosteal incision

Triceps brachii m., lateral head

Superficial pectoral m.

Brachialis m.

Brachiocephalicus m.

Radial n.

Anconeus m.

Extensor carpi radialis m.

A

C

139

Approach to the Distal Shaft of the Humerus Through a Craniolateral Incision *continued*

DESCRIPTION OF THE PROCEDURE *continued*

D. The superficial pectoral muscle is elevated at its insertion on the humerus as necessary to allow cranial retraction. The brachialis muscle is freed from the bone by blunt dissection and is retracted caudally with the triceps and the radial nerve.

E. To obtain better exposure of the distal portion of the bone, the lateral head of the triceps brachii muscle can be retracted caudally and the brachialis muscle and radial nerve retracted cranially.

CLOSURE

Interrupted sutures are placed between external fascia of the brachialis and brachiocephalicus/superficial pectoral muscles. Deep brachial fascia is attached to the triceps, and subcutaneous tissue and skin are closed in layers.

COMMENTS

Great care must be taken at all times to protect the radial nerve.

Plate 32

Approach to the Distal Shaft of the Humerus Through a Craniolateral Incision *continued*

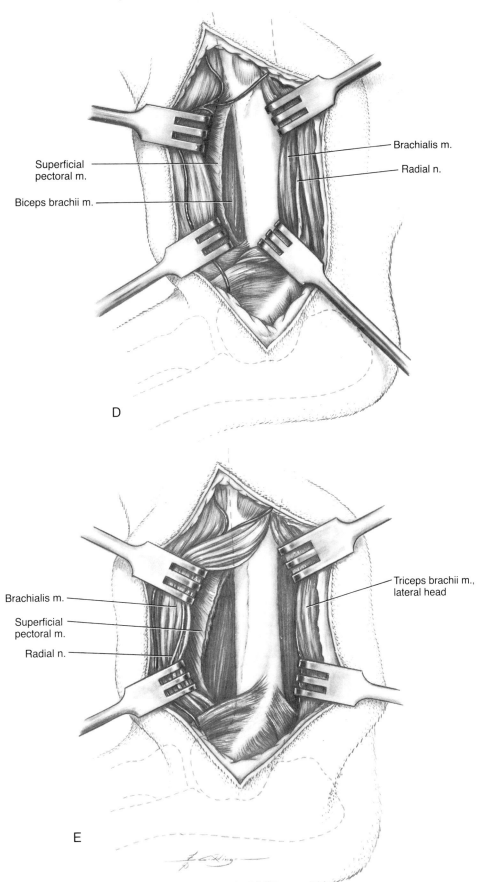

Superficial pectoral m.

Biceps brachii m.

Brachialis m.

Radial n.

D

Brachialis m.

Superficial pectoral m.

Radial n.

Triceps brachii m., lateral head

E

Approach to the Distal Shaft and Supracondylar Region of the Humerus Through a Medial Incision

Based on a Procedure of Brinker[4]

INDICATION

Open reduction of fractures of the humerus at midshaft or distally.

ALTERNATIVE/COMBINATION APPROACHES

Plates 31 and 41

DESCRIPTION OF THE PROCEDURE

A. The skin incision extends from the medial epicondyle proximally along the cranial border of the humerus to the midshaft of the bone.

B. The skin is undermined and the subcutaneous fat is elevated sufficiently to allow visualization of the brachial and collateral ulnar vessels. The ulnar and median nerves that accompany these vessels are not yet visible; they lie slightly deeper. An incision is made in the deep fascia directly over the distal shaft of the humerus and between the blood vessels. It will be necessary to continue the incision proximally over the vessels.

C. Blunt dissection of the subfascial fat will expose the underlying structures.

Plate 33

Approach to the Distal Shaft and Supracondylar Region of the Humerus Through a Medial Incision

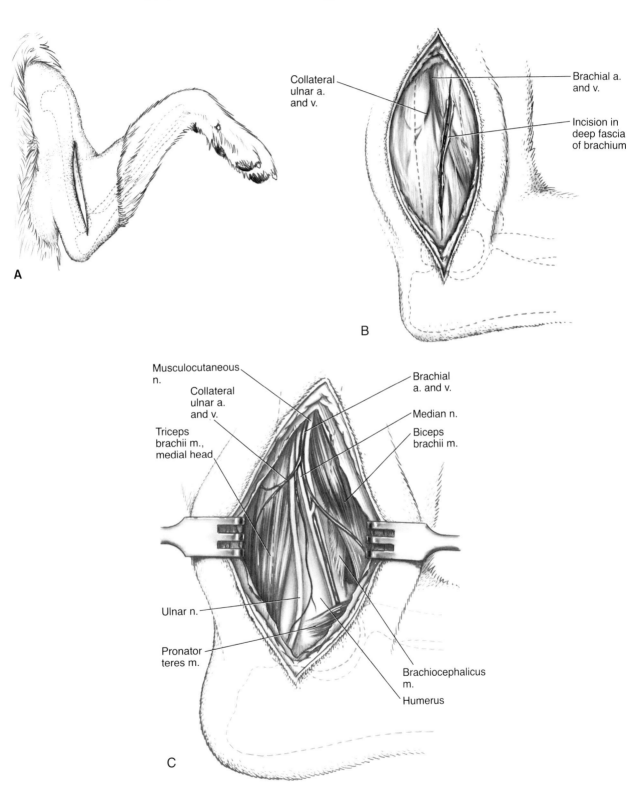

A

B

Collateral ulnar a. and v.

Brachial a. and v.

Incision in deep fascia of brachium

C

Musculocutaneous n.

Collateral ulnar a. and v.

Triceps brachii m., medial head

Brachial a. and v.

Median n.

Biceps brachii m.

Ulnar n.

Pronator teres m.

Brachiocephalicus m.

Humerus

Approach to the Distal Shaft and Supracondylar Region of the Humerus Through a Medial Incision *continued*

DESCRIPTION OF THE PROCEDURE *continued*

D. The manner in which the vessels and the nerves are mobilized depends on the area of the bone that is to be exposed. The method illustrated is used when the extreme distal portion of the bone is involved. If the proximal portion of the exposed area is of more interest, the vessels and nerves may be freed and retracted caudally with the triceps and the collateral ulnar vessels.

   The biceps brachii and triceps brachii muscles are elevated from the shaft of the bone. The periosteal branches of blood vessels are ligated or coagulated as required. Subperiosteal elevation of a portion of the insertion of the superficial pectoral and brachiocephalicus muscles is necessary to fully expose the cranial surface of the bone.

E. In the *cat,* retraction of the neurovascular components is complicated by the passage of the brachial artery and median nerve through the supratrochlear foramen of the humerus. Note also the short part of the medial head of the triceps brachii muscle running caudal to the medial aspect of the humeral condyle and inserting on the medial side of the olecranon process. If this muscle is elevated to expose a fracture line, care must be taken to protect the ulnar nerve deep to it.

CLOSURE

The deep fascia, subcutaneous tissues, and skin are closed in separate layers.

COMMENTS

If great care is taken to protect the vessels and nerves, some exposure of the shaft proximal to the midportion can be obtained. This exposure is sufficient to allow insertion of the proximal screws in a bone plate. Better exposure is detailed in Plate 31.

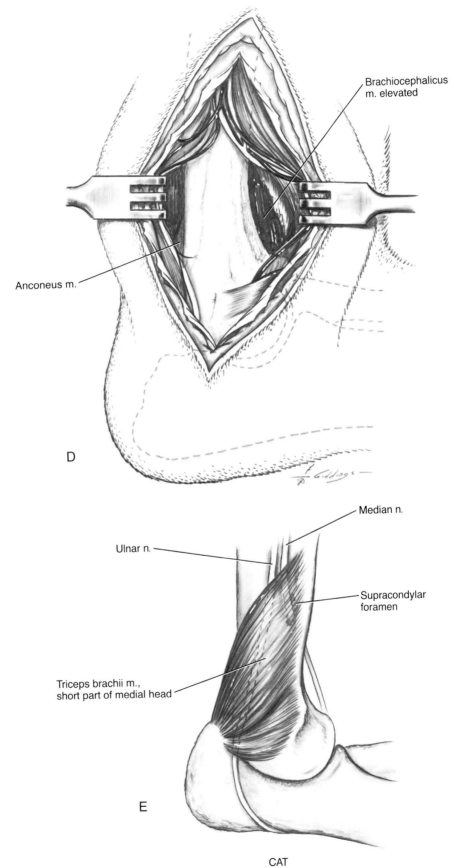

Brachiocephalicus m. elevated

Anconeus m.

D

Median n.

Ulnar n.

Supracondylar foramen

Triceps brachii m., short part of medial head

E

CAT

Approach to the Lateral Aspect of the Humeral Condyle and Epicondyle

Based on a Procedure of Turner and Hohn[40]

INDICATIONS

1. Open reduction of fractures of the humeral capitulum.
2. Open reduction of lateral elbow luxation.

ALTERNATIVE/COMBINATION APPROACHES

Plates 35, 36, and 39

DESCRIPTION OF THE PROCEDURE

A. The skin incision extends along the lower fourth of the humerus and crosses the joint to end distally on the ulna. The incision passes over or slightly caudal to the lateral epicondyle. The subcutaneous fascia is incised on the same line.

B. As the skin and subcutaneous fascia are retracted, the deep brachial and antebrachial fascia and the lateral head of the triceps muscle are exposed. An incision is made through the deep fascia near the cranial border of the triceps and is continued distally over the extensor muscles.

C. Retraction of the fascia exposes the condylar region of the humerus. Although it is proximal to the main area of exposure, it is well to note the location of the radial nerve. An incision is started distally in the intermuscular septum between the extensor carpi radialis and the common digital extensor muscles. This incision continues proximally into the periosteal origin of the distal half of the extensor carpi radialis muscle.

Plate 34

Approach to the Lateral Aspect of the Humeral Condyle and Epicondyle

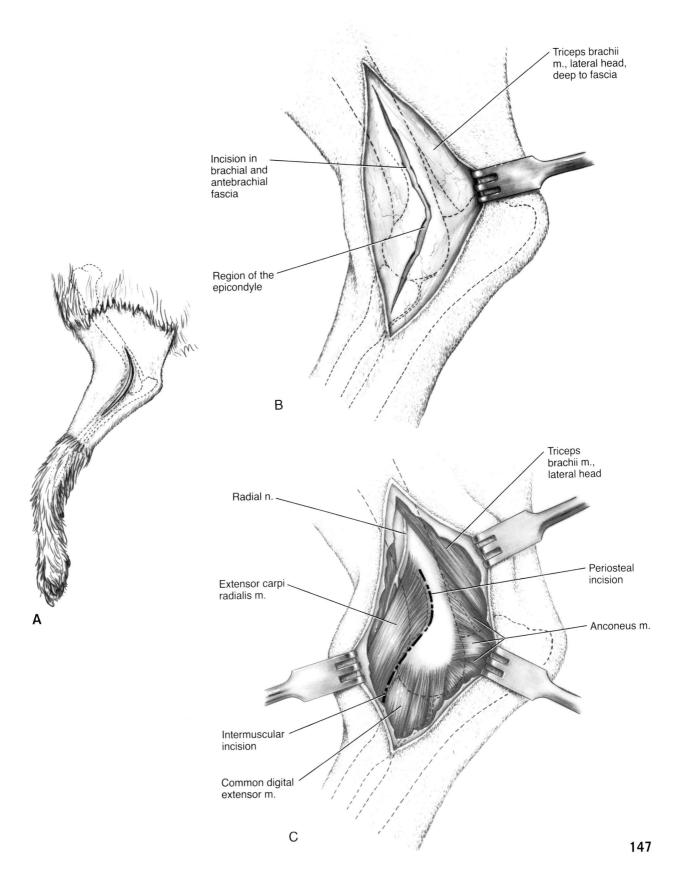

Triceps brachii m., lateral head, deep to fascia

Incision in brachial and antebrachial fascia

Region of the epicondyle

B

Triceps brachii m., lateral head

Radial n.

Periosteal incision

Extensor carpi radialis m.

Anconeus m.

Intermuscular incision

Common digital extensor m.

A

C

Approach to the Lateral Aspect of the Humeral Condyle and Epicondyle *continued*

DESCRIPTION OF THE PROCEDURE *continued*

D. The extensor carpi radialis muscle is elevated from the bone and underlying joint capsule, and the capsule is opened with an L-shaped incision. Care must be taken to protect the cartilage of the condyle.

E. Retraction of the joint capsule reveals the humeral condyle.

CLOSURE

The joint capsule is closed with interrupted sutures. A continuous pattern can be used in the intermuscular incision. If there is no tissue available to reattach the extensor carpi radialis to the humerus, the muscle can be sutured to the external fascia of the anconeus muscle. The brachial and antebrachial fascia is closed with a continuous pattern.

Plate 34

Approach to the Lateral Aspect of the Humeral Condyle and Epicondyle *continued*

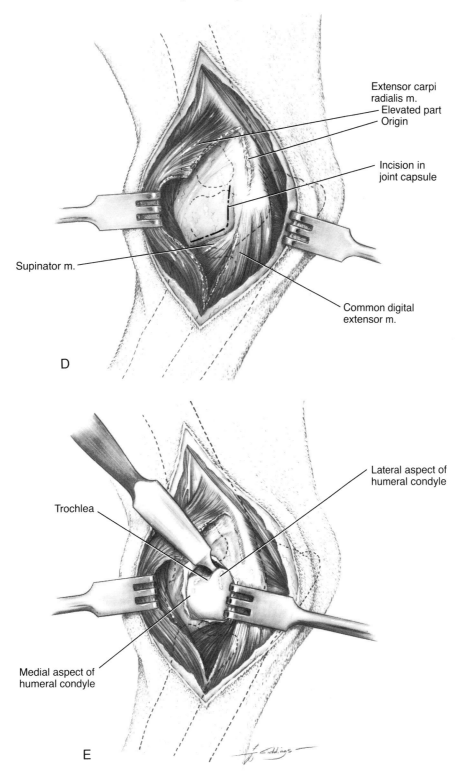

Extensor carpi radialis m.
Elevated part
Origin

Incision in joint capsule

Supinator m.

Common digital extensor m.

D

Lateral aspect of humeral condyle

Trochlea

Medial aspect of humeral condyle

E

Approach to the Lateral Humeroulnar Part of the Elbow Joint

Based on a Procedure of Snavely and Hohn[37]

INDICATIONS

1. Excision or fixation of ununited anconeal process.
2. Open reduction of lateral elbow luxation.

ALTERNATIVE/COMBINATION APPROACHES

Plates 33, 34, and 36

DESCRIPTION OF THE PROCEDURE

A. The skin incision is centered on the lateral humeral epicondyle, which is easily palpated. The incision curves to follow the lateral epicondylar crest and the proximal radius.

B. Subcutaneous fascia is incised on the same line as the skin. The fascia of the brachium is incised along the cranial border of the lateral head of the triceps brachii to its insertion on the olecranon.

Plate 35

Approach to the Lateral Humeroulnar Part of the Elbow Joint

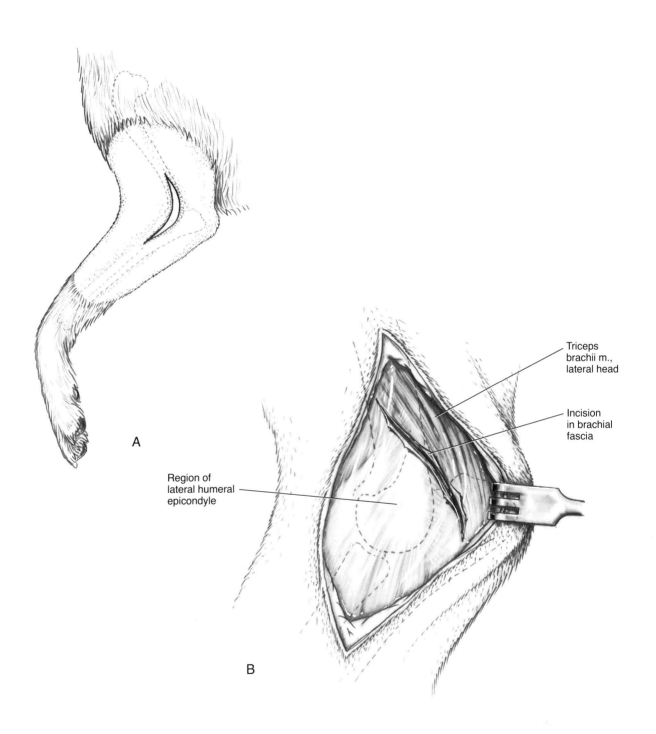

A

B

Triceps
brachii m.,
lateral head

Incision
in brachial
fascia

Region of
lateral humeral
epicondyle

Approach to the Lateral Humeroulnar Part of the Elbow Joint *continued*

DESCRIPTION OF THE PROCEDURE *continued*

C. Elevation of the triceps brachii exposes the anconeus muscle, which is incised at its periosteal origin on the lateral epicondylar crest.

D. Subperiosteal elevation of the origin of the anconeus muscle exposes the caudolateral compartment of the elbow and the anconeal process of the olecranon.

CLOSURE

The origin of the anconeal muscle is sutured to the origins of the extensor muscles of the antebrachium. The fascia of the triceps brachii, subcutaneous fascia, and skin are closed in separate layers.

Plate 35

Approach to the Lateral Humeroulnar Part
of the Elbow Joint *continued*

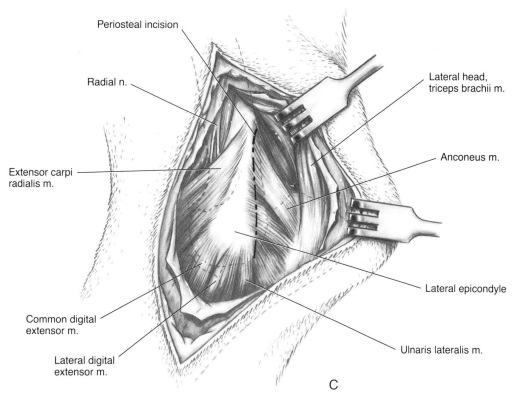

Periosteal incision

Radial n.

Extensor carpi
radialis m.

Common digital
extensor m.

Lateral digital
extensor m.

Lateral head,
triceps brachii m.

Anconeus m.

Lateral epicondyle

Ulnaris lateralis m.

C

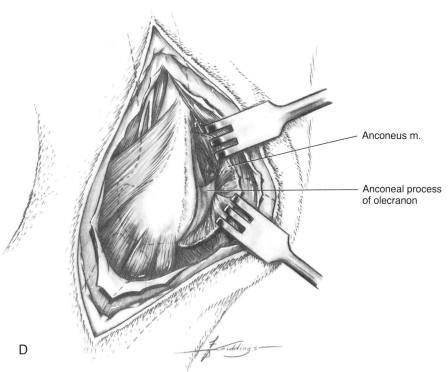

Anconeus m.

Anconeal process
of olecranon

D

Approach to the Supracondylar Region of the Humerus and the Caudal Humeroulnar Part of the Elbow Joint

Based on a procedure of Chalman and Slocum[1]

INDICATIONS

1. Reduction of supracondylar or lateral condylar fractures of the humerus.
2. Reduction of lateral luxation of the elbow joint.
3. Excision or fixation of ununited anconeal process.

ALTERNATIVE/COMBINATION APPROACHES

Plates 33, 34, 35, 37, and 38

DESCRIPTION OF THE PROCEDURE

A. The skin incision starts just distal to the midshaft of the humerus and follows the caudal edge of the bone distally. At the level of the lateral humeral epicondyle, the incision curves between the epicondylar crest and the tuber olecrani and continues distally along the ulna.

B. Subcutaneous fat and fascia are incised on the same line as the skin and then elevated from the deep brachial fascia to allow wide retraction of the skin margins. An incision is made in the deep brachial fascia over the division between the long and lateral heads of the triceps brachii muscle. This incision is slightly caudal and roughly parallel to the shaft of the humerus. Distally, it extends into the tendon of insertion of the lateral head of the triceps brachii muscle on the tuber olecrani, where a few millimeters of tendon are left on the olecranon to facilitate closure.

Plate 36

Approach to the Supracondylar Region of the Humerus and the Caudal Humeroulnar Part of the Elbow Joint

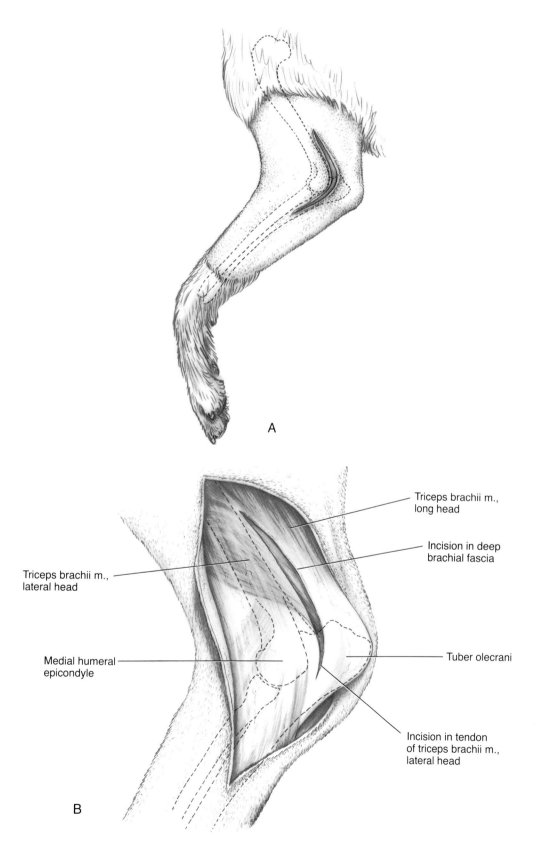

Triceps brachii m.,
long head

Incision in deep
brachial fascia

Triceps brachii m.,
lateral head

Tuber olecrani

Medial humeral
epicondyle

Incision in tendon
of triceps brachii m.,
lateral head

A

B

Approach to the Supracondylar Region of the Humerus and the Caudal Humeroulnar Part of the Elbow Joint *continued*

DESCRIPTION OF THE PROCEDURE *continued*

C. The separation between the heads of the triceps is developed by blunt dissection; it is limited by the collateral radial vessels and a muscular branch of the radial nerve proximally and by the tuber olecrani distally. Blunt dissection is also used to separate the long head of the triceps brachii muscle from the anconeus muscle. The periosteal insertion of the anconeus muscle is incised on the ulna and tuber olecrani and on the medial epicondylar crest.

D. Retraction of the elevated anconeus muscle and the long head of the triceps brachii muscle exposes the anconeal process, the lateral aspect of the humeral condyle, and the supracondylar region of the humerus.

CLOSURE

The anconeus muscle is sutured to fascia and remnants of periosteum on the medial epicondylar crest and ulna. The deep antebrachial fascia and tendon of insertion of the triceps brachii muscle are closed in the next layer. Subcutaneous tissues and skin are closed in two layers.

COMMENTS

This approach is particularly useful for supracondylar fractures, where it may eliminate the need for a combined medial and lateral approach. A variation is elevation of the anconeus muscle from the lateral epicondylar crest, similar to that shown in Plate 35D.

Plate 36

Approach to the Supracondylar Region of the Humerus and the Caudal Humeroulnar Part of the Elbow Joint *continued*

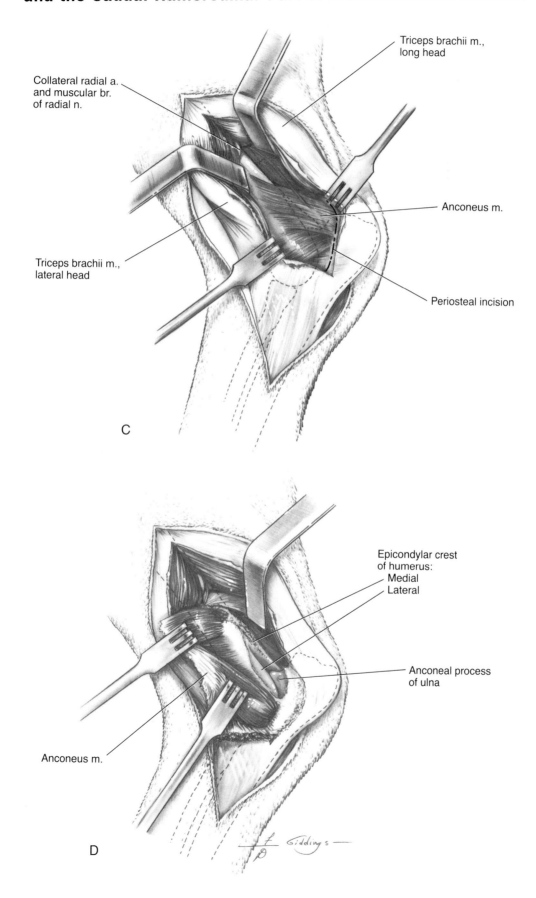

Triceps brachii m., long head

Collateral radial a. and muscular br. of radial n.

Anconeus m.

Triceps brachii m., lateral head

Periosteal incision

C

Epicondylar crest of humerus:
 Medial
 Lateral

Anconeal process of ulna

Anconeus m.

D

157

Approach to the Humeroulnar Part of the Elbow Joint by Osteotomy of the Tuber Olecrani

Based on a Procedure of Mostosky, Cholvin, and Brinker[24]

INDICATIONS

1. Open reduction of fractures of the condylar and supracondylar region of the humerus.
2. Open reduction of chronic luxations of the elbow joint.
3. Exploration of the caudal compartment of the elbow joint.

ALTERNATIVE/COMBINATION APPROACHES

Plates 31, 32, 33, 34, and 36

DESCRIPTION OF THE PROCEDURE

A. A skin incision is made slightly lateral to the caudal midline of the leg. The incision extends from the distal third of the humerus to the proximal third of the ulna, and crosses the elbow joint between the olecranon process and the lateral epicondyle.

B. Subcutaneous fat and fascia are incised and then widely undermined to allow retraction of the cranial skin margin beyond the lateral epicondyle and the caudal margin medial to the olecranon process. An incision is made in the fascia of the triceps brachii along the cranial border of the lateral head to allow elevation of its tendon from the olecranon.

C. The leg is elevated and the elbow flexed to allow dissection of the medial side of the joint.

Plate 37

Approach to the Humeroulnar Part of the Elbow Joint by Osteotomy of the Tuber Olecrani

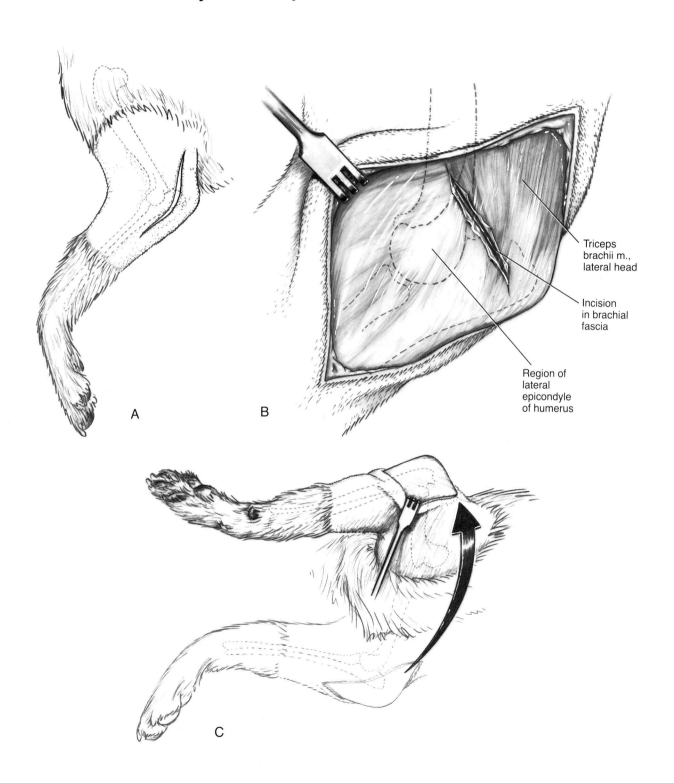

Triceps
brachii m.,
lateral head

Incision
in brachial
fascia

Region of
lateral
epicondyle
of humerus

A

B

C

Approach to the Humeroulnar Part of the Elbow Joint by Osteotomy of the Tuber Olecrani *continued*

DESCRIPTION OF THE PROCEDURE *continued*

D. Undermining of the subcutaneous fat and fascia continues around the joint to the medial side, until the caudal skin margin can be retracted beyond the medial epicondyle. After incising the triceps fascia, the cranial border of the medial head of the triceps is undermined from proximal to the medial condyle to the olecranon. The ulnar nerve and collateral ulnar vessels lie parallel to the cranial border of the medial head and deep to it, under the antebrachial fascia (see Figure 33C). The nerve and vessels should be identified and protected throughout the procedure by retracting them distally.

When operating on the *cat,* refer at this point to Part E of Plate 33.

E. A Gigli wire saw is pulled between the two fascial incisions, cranial to the tendon of the triceps brachii on the olecranon, resting on the bone in the notch between the olecranon and anconeal processes. Care must be exercised at this point to be certain the ulnar nerve and collateral ulnar vessels are free from the wire. The olecranon process is then osteotomized with the wire saw at approximately a 45° angle to the shaft of the ulna. A power saw can also be used, but osteotomes should be avoided. The bone is so hard that it shatters easily.

Plate 37

Approach to the Humeroulnar Part of the Elbow Joint by Osteotomy of the Tuber Olecrani *continued*

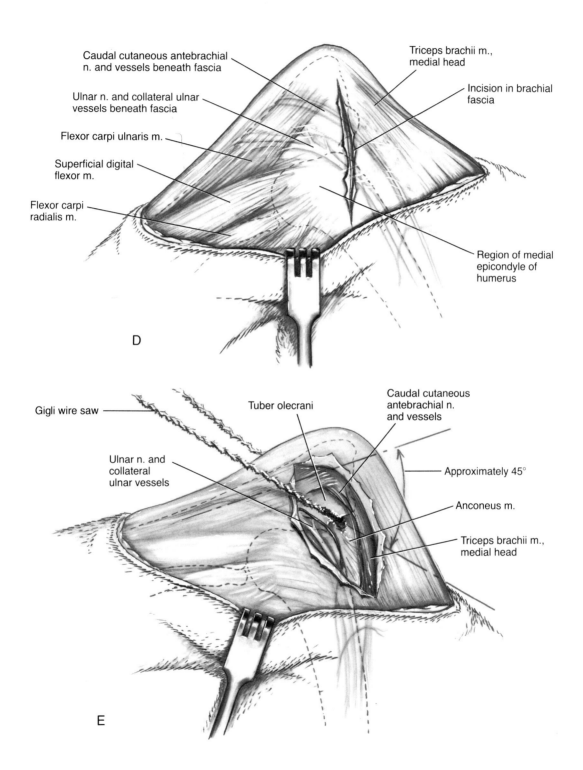

Caudal cutaneous antebrachial n. and vessels beneath fascia

Ulnar n. and collateral ulnar vessels beneath fascia

Flexor carpi ulnaris m.

Superficial digital flexor m.

Flexor carpi radialis m.

Triceps brachii m., medial head

Incision in brachial fascia

Region of medial epicondyle of humerus

D

Gigli wire saw

Ulnar n. and collateral ulnar vessels

Tuber olecrani

Caudal cutaneous antebrachial n. and vessels

Approximately 45°

Anconeus m.

Triceps brachii m., medial head

E

Approach to the Humeroulnar Part of the Elbow Joint by Osteotomy of the Tuber Olecrani *continued*

DESCRIPTION OF THE PROCEDURE *continued*

F. The olecranon process with the attached triceps brachii muscle can now be reflected proximally to reveal the entire caudal surface of the joint. If the anconeus muscle is intact, an incision is made through the muscle and the underlying joint capsule near their attachments from just proximal to the medial aspect of the humeral condyle, continuing distally onto the olecranon. If possible, the branch of the collateral ulnar vessel that penetrates the muscle is preserved.

G. Maximum exposure of the intraarticular area is gained by complete flexion of the joint and retraction of the anconeus muscle.

CLOSURE

No attempt is made to close the incision in the anconeus. The olecranon process is reattached by the tension band wire technique (Figure 23). The cranial borders of the triceps are sutured to the surrounding deep fascia, and subcutaneous sutures are used to pull the fat and fascia together and to take some of the tension off the skin sutures.

Plate 37

Approach to the Humeroulnar Part of the Elbow Joint by Osteotomy of the Tuber Olecrani *continued*

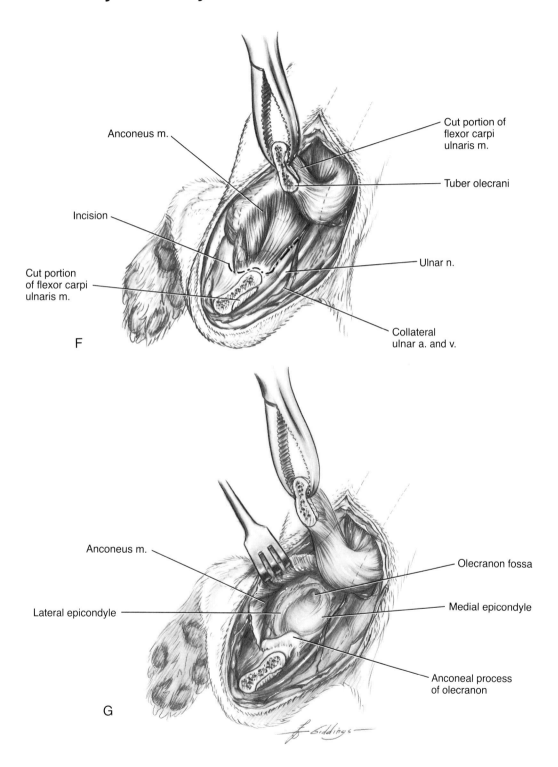

Anconeus m.

Cut portion of flexor carpi ulnaris m.

Tuber olecrani

Incision

Ulnar n.

Cut portion of flexor carpi ulnaris m.

Collateral ulnar a. and v.

F

Anconeus m.

Olecranon fossa

Lateral epicondyle

Medial epicondyle

Anconeal process of olecranon

G

Approach to the Elbow Joint by Osteotomy of the Proximal Ulnar Diaphysis

Based on a Procedure of Lenehan and Nunamaker[21]

INDICATIONS

1. Open reduction of multiple intraarticular fractures of the humeral condyle.
2. Open reduction of luxations of the elbow joint.
3. Exploration of multiple compartments of the elbow joint.

ALTERNATIVE/COMBINATION APPROACHES

Plates 34, 37, 41, and 44

DESCRIPTION OF THE PROCEDURE

A. The skin incision starts proximally at the level of the lateral epicondyle, halfway between it and the tuber olecrani. The incision curves distally following the lateral epicondylar crest, ending at the junction of the proximal and middle thirds of the ulna lateral to that bone.

B. Two incisions are made in the deep antebrachial fascia covering the muscles and ulna. The lateral incision runs between the ulna and the caudal border of the ulnaris lateralis muscle distally and through the insertion of the anconeus muscle on the tuber olecrani proximally. The medial incision is between the flexor carpi ulnaris and the ulna.

C. The anconeus and flexor carpi ulnaris muscles are subperiosteally elevated from the ulna. Retraction of the muscles will reveal the ulnar nerve and collateral ulnar vessels medially, running on the deep surface of the flexor muscles. The cranial interosseous vessels and interosseous nerve cross the field between the radius and ulna. The ulnar head of the deep digital flexor and the abductor pollicis longus muscles are subperiosteally elevated from the ulna to reveal the interosseous membrane and ligament. The ulnar collateral ligament (caudal crus) and annular ligament are incised on the lateral aspect of the radioulnar joint.

Plate 38

Approach to the Elbow Joint by Osteotomy of the Proximal Ulnar Diaphysis

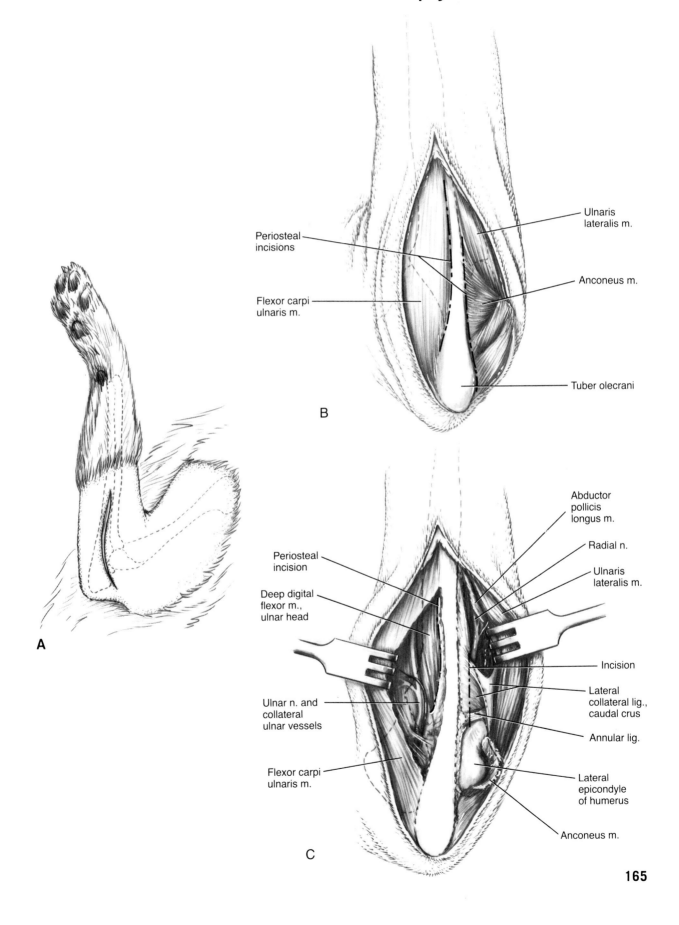

A

B

Periosteal incisions

Flexor carpi ulnaris m.

Ulnaris lateralis m.

Anconeus m.

Tuber olecrani

C

Periosteal incision

Deep digital flexor m., ulnar head

Ulnar n. and collateral ulnar vessels

Flexor carpi ulnaris m.

Abductor pollicis longus m.

Radial n.

Ulnaris lateralis m.

Incision

Lateral collateral lig., caudal crus

Annular lig.

Lateral epicondyle of humerus

Anconeus m.

165

Approach to the Elbow Joint by Osteotomy of the Proximal Ulnar Diaphysis *continued*

DESCRIPTION OF THE PROCEDURE *continued*

D. Osteotomy of the ulna is performed just proximal to the interosseous ligament, taking care to protect the interosseous vessels and nerve. The osteotomy can be performed with a Gigli wire saw, as illustrated, or with a power saw. An osteotome should not be used, because it tends to fragment the ulna.

E. Medial rotation of the proximal ulnar segment exposes the humeral condyle and radial head. Transection of the olecranon ligament will allow additional rotation of the ulna if required. Distraction of the humeroradial joint allows inspection of the articular surface of the radius, and extreme flexion of the joint exposes the humeral condyle fully.

CLOSURE

The proximal ulnar segment is reduced and fixed with one or two Steinmann pins or Kirschner wires driven from the tuber olecrani. Interfragmentary compression is supplied with a figure-of-8 wire (see Figure 23). No attempt is made to repair the ulnar collateral or annular ligament. Adequate stability of the elbow is afforded by the intact cranial crus of the collateral ligament and the muscles. The superficial fascia of the flexor carpi ulnaris is sutured to the fascia of the ulnaris lateralis and anconeus muscles. Proximally, the anconeus muscle is sutured to remnants of periosteum and fascia.

COMMENTS

Passive range of motion exercises and early weight bearing should be encouraged to restore function to the joint. Although this approach seems radical, it is less traumatic than combining approaches if generous exposure is needed.

Plate 38

Approach to the Elbow Joint by Osteotomy of the Proximal Ulnar Diaphysis *continued*

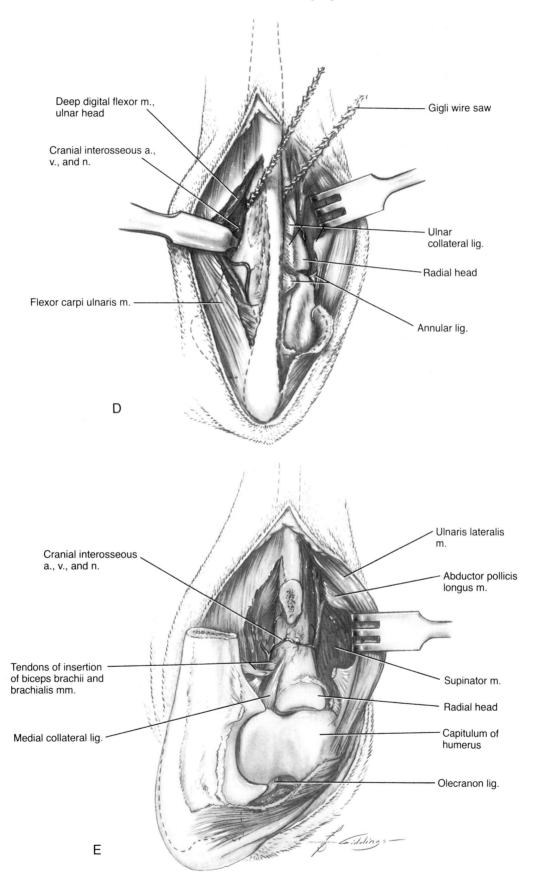

Deep digital flexor m., ulnar head

Cranial interosseous a., v., and n.

Gigli wire saw

Flexor carpi ulnaris m.

Ulnar collateral lig.

Radial head

Annular lig.

D

Cranial interosseous a., v., and n.

Ulnaris lateralis m.

Abductor pollicis longus m.

Tendons of insertion of biceps brachii and brachialis mm.

Medial collateral lig.

Supinator m.

Radial head

Capitulum of humerus

Olecranon lig.

E

Approach to the Head of the Radius and Lateral Parts of the Elbow Joint

INDICATIONS

1. Open reduction of lateral luxations of the head of the radius.
2. Open reduction of fractures of the head of the radius.

ALTERNATIVE/COMBINATION APPROACHES

Plates 34, 35, 36, 37, 38, 40, and 47

DESCRIPTION OF THE PROCEDURE

A. The curved incision commences proximal to the lateral humeral epicondyle, crosses the joint following the lateral surface of the radius, and ends at the proximal fourth of the radius. Subcutaneous fascia is incised on the same line.

B. After retraction of the skin and subcutaneous fascia, the deeper lying brachial and antebrachial fascia is incised on a similar line.

C. Incision and retraction of the fascia of the triceps brachii allows retraction of the lateral head of the triceps muscle and incision of the origin of the anconeus muscle along the lateral epicondylar crest. The tendon of origin and proximal portion of the ulnaris lateralis muscle are isolated and the tendon cut, leaving enough tendon proximally to allow suturing.

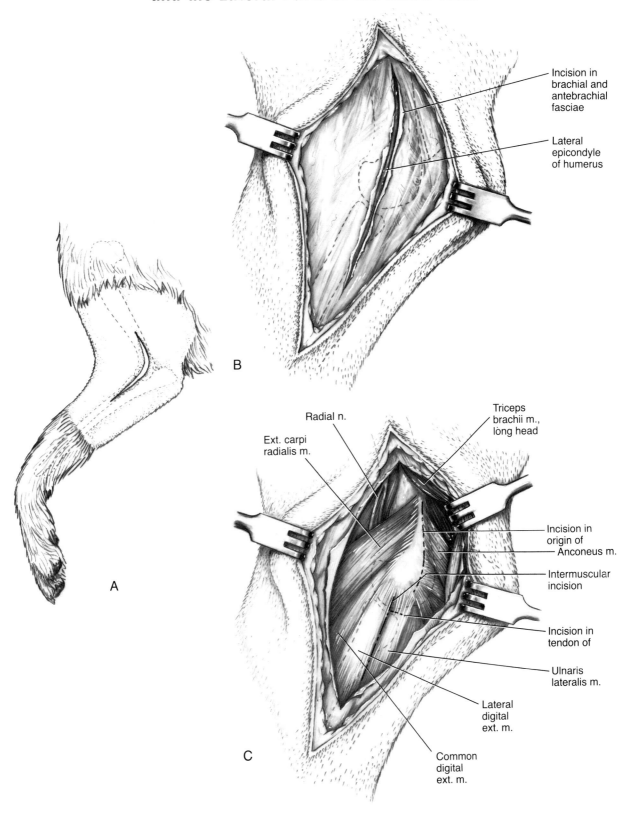

Plate 39

Approach to the Head of the Radius and the Lateral Parts of the Elbow Joint

Incision in brachial and antebrachial fasciae

Lateral epicondyle of humerus

Radial n.

Ext. carpi radialis m.

Triceps brachii m., long head

Incision in origin of Anconeus m.

Intermuscular incision

Incision in tendon of

Ulnaris lateralis m.

Lateral digital ext. m.

Common digital ext. m.

A

B

C

Approach to the Head of the Radius and Lateral Parts of the Elbow Joint *continued*

DESCRIPTION OF THE PROCEDURE *continued*

D. Subperiosteal elevation of the anconeus muscle exposes the caudolateral humeroulnar joint compartment.

E. The remaining extensor muscles are elevated with a Hohmann retractor. The tip of the retractor must be kept on the bone to avoid damage to the radial nerve. Transection of the annular and collateral ligaments may be necessary to gain adequate exposure of the head of the radius.

CLOSURE

Transected portions of the collateral ligament are sutured to the remaining portions of the ligament. The tendon of the ulnaris lateralis muscle is reattached with a modified Bunnell-Mayer or locking-loop stitch (see Figure 21). The origin of the anconeus muscle is sewn to the origins of the extensor muscles and the cranial edge of the triceps brachii is attached to the brachial fascia. The two fascial layers and skin are closed routinely, in separate layers.

Plate 39

Approach to the Head of the Radius
and the Lateral Parts of the Elbow Joint *continued*

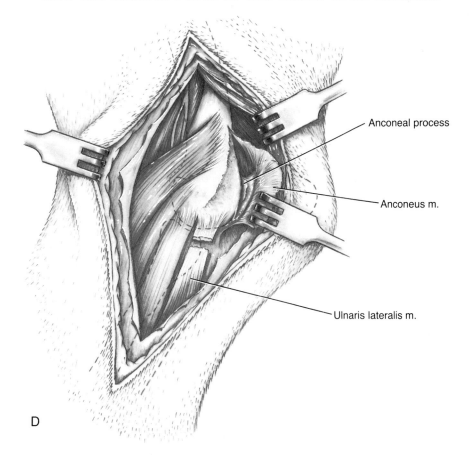

Anconeal process

Anconeus m.

Ulnaris lateralis m.

D

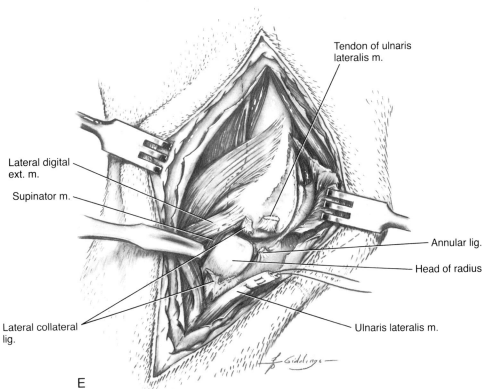

Tendon of ulnaris
lateralis m.

Lateral digital
ext. m.

Supinator m.

Annular lig.

Head of radius

Lateral collateral
lig.

Ulnaris lateralis m.

E

171

Approach to the Head of the Radius and Humeroradial Part of the Elbow Joint by Osteotomy of the Lateral Humeral Epicondyle

Based on a Procedure of Hohn[17]

INDICATIONS

1. Open reduction of lateral luxation of the head of the radius.
2. Open reduction of fractures of the head of the radius.

ALTERNATIVE/COMBINATION APPROACHES

Plates 34, 35, 36, 37, 38, 39, and 47

DESCRIPTION OF THE PROCEDURE

A. The curved incision commences proximal to the lateral humeral epicondyle, crosses the joint following the lateral surface of the radius, and ends at the proximal fourth of the radius. Subcutaneous and deep antebrachial fascia is incised on the same line.

B. Antebrachial and intermuscular fasciae are incised from the cranioventral borders of the lateral head of the triceps brachii distally, along a line that separates the extensor carpi radialis from the common digital extensor muscle. A similar incision is made between the anconeus and ulnaris lateralis muscles. These incisions are deepened to completely free the three enclosed extensor muscles from the underlying bone. If the epicondyle is to be reattached by a lag screw (see "Closure" below), a suitable glide and tap hole should be drilled now, just distal to the epicondyle.

Plate 40

Approach to the Head of the Radius and Humeroradial Part of the Elbow Joint by Osteotomy of the Lateral Humeral Condyle

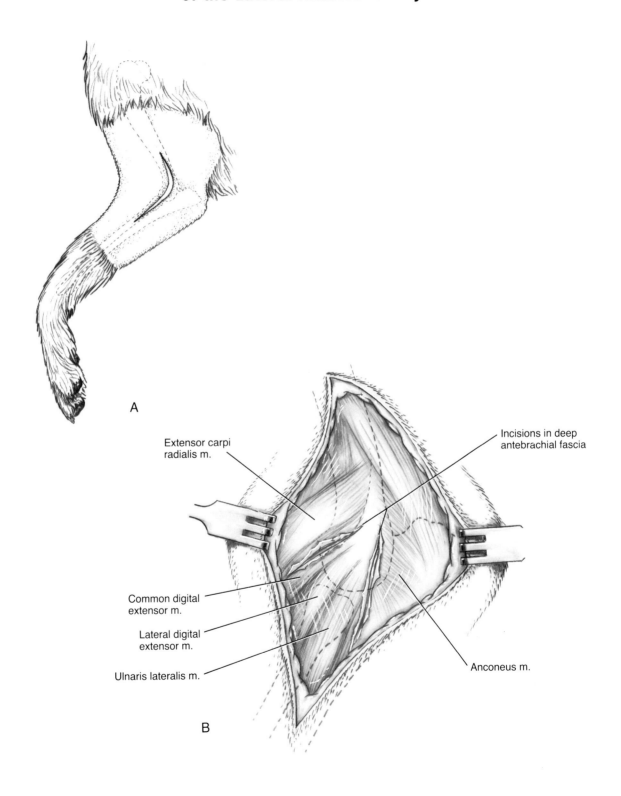

A

Extensor carpi
radialis m.

Incisions in deep
antebrachial fascia

Common digital
extensor m.

Lateral digital
extensor m.

Ulnaris lateralis m.

Anconeus m.

B

Approach to the Head of the Radius and Humeroradial Part of the Elbow Joint by Osteotomy of the Lateral Humeral Epicondyle *continued*

DESCRIPTION OF THE PROCEDURE *continued*

C. The lateral humeral epicondyle is osteotomized so as to include the origins of the three extensor muscles. The angle of the osteotomy from a cranial perspective is shown in Part C1. No articular cartilage should be included in the osteotomy.

D. Retraction of the osteotomized epicondyle with attached collateral ligaments and extensor muscles is possible after incision of the joint capsule where necessary. Elevation of the supinator muscle will further expose the head of the radius. Care should be taken to protect the radial nerve, which crosses under the deep surface of the supinator muscle.

CLOSURE

The humeral epicondyle is reattached to its origin by a lag screw or pins and tension band wire (see Figures 23 and 24). Incisions in the intermuscular septa, deep antebrachial fascia, subcutaneous fascia, and skin are each closed in separate layers.

COMMENTS

This approach is very similar to that shown in Plate 39. Slightly better exposure of the radial head is gained here. The choice of tenotomy or osteotomy is primarily a matter of personal preference. Simultaneous access to the caudal compartment of the elbow joint can be gained by elevation of the origin of the anconeus muscle (see Plate 35).

Plate 40

Approach to the Head of the Radius and Humeroradial Part of the Elbow Joint by Osteotomy of the Lateral Humeral Condyle *continued*

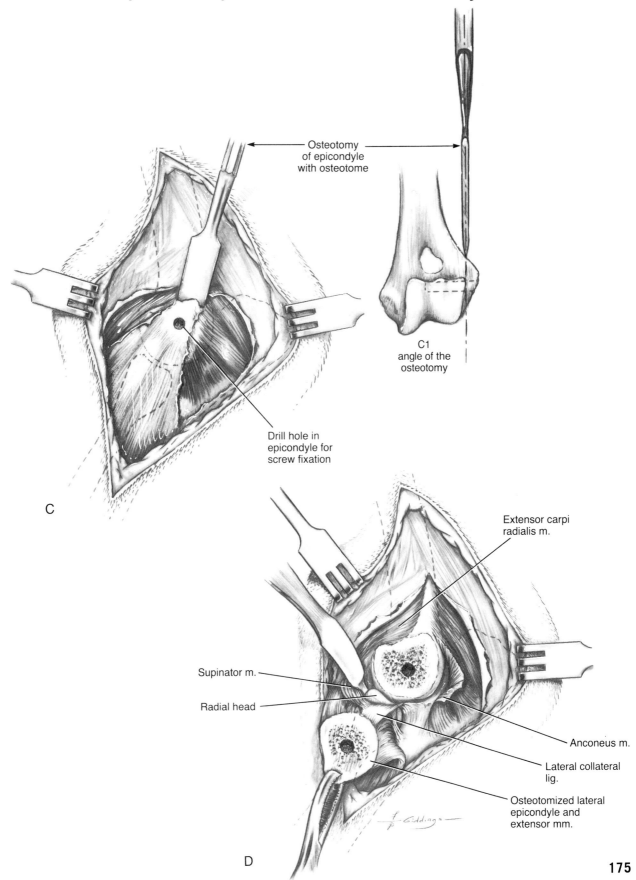

Osteotomy of epicondyle with osteotome

C1 angle of the osteotomy

Drill hole in epicondyle for screw fixation

C

Extensor carpi radialis m.

Supinator m.

Radial head

Anconeus m.

Lateral collateral lig.

Osteotomized lateral epicondyle and extensor mm.

D

Approach to the Medial Humeral Epicondyle

INDICATIONS

1. Reduction of fractures of the medial aspect of the humeral condyle.
2. Reduction of medial luxations of the elbow joint.

ALTERNATIVE/COMBINATION APPROACHES

Plates 31, 33, 42, and 43

DESCRIPTION OF THE PROCEDURE

A. The skin incision is centered on the medial humeral epicondyle and follows the humeral shaft proximally and the shaft of the ulna distally. It may be useful to lengthen the incision in some cases. The subcutaneous fat and fascia are incised on the same line and retracted with the skin.

B. The deep antebrachial fascia is incised in each direction from the epicondyle on the same line as the skin. Be aware of the neurovascular tissues deep to the fascia, as illustrated in Part C.

C. Retraction of the deep fascia and clearing of areolar tissue will expose the epicondyle and the attached flexor muscle group. Dissection in the craniomedial direction must take into account the median nerve and brachial vessels, whereas the ulnar nerve and collateral ulnar vessels lie caudolateral to the epicondyle.

CLOSURE

The deep antebrachial and brachial fascia is closed, followed by closure of the subcutaneous tissues and then closure of the skin.

COMMENTS

This approach forms the basis for several other approaches to the medial side of the elbow joint and will be cross-referenced in those approaches.

Plate 41

Approach to the Medial Humeral Epicondyle

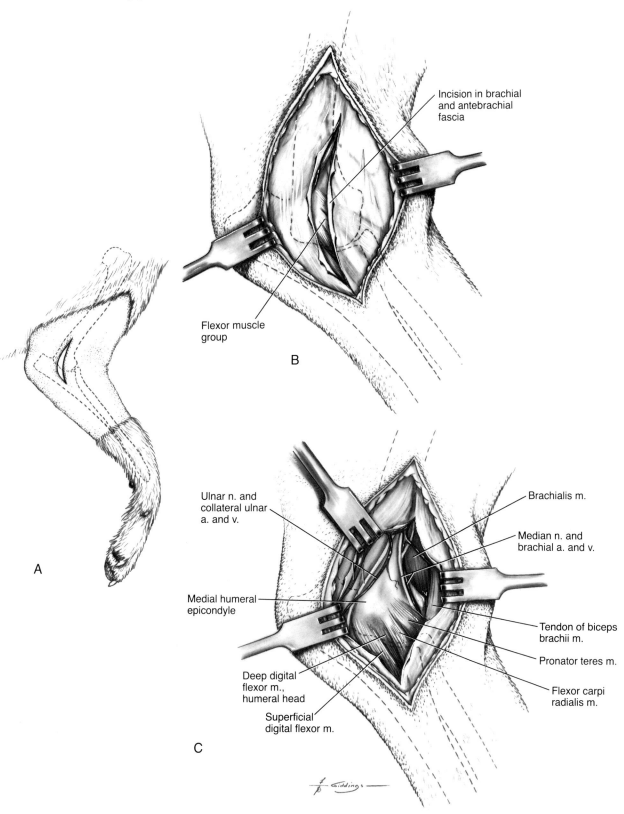

Incision in brachial and antebrachial fascia

Flexor muscle group

B

A

Ulnar n. and collateral ulnar a. and v.

Brachialis m.

Median n. and brachial a. and v.

Medial humeral epicondyle

Tendon of biceps brachii m.

Pronator teres m.

Deep digital flexor m., humeral head

Flexor carpi radialis m.

Superficial digital flexor m.

C

Approach to the Medial Aspect of the Humeral Condyle and the Medial Coronoid Process of the Ulna by an Intermuscular Incision

Based on a Procedure of Probst, et al.[30]

INDICATION

Exploration of the medial elbow joint for osteochondritis dissecans and fragmented medial coronoid process.

ALTERNATIVE/COMBINATION APPROACH

Plate 43

DESCRIPTION OF THE PROCEDURE

A. This approach starts similarly to that shown in Plate 41, but the skin incision extends further distally. Deep antebrachial fascia is incised on the same line as the skin and retracted to expose the flexor muscle group, as in Plate 41, Parts B and C. Protect the ulnar nerve during the fascial incision and elevation.

B. The intermuscular septum between the flexor carpi radialis and deep digital flexor muscles is incised following ligation or coagulation of the intermuscular vessels. The division between these muscles is often not very distinct, but can be found by blunt dissection. The intermuscular incision can alternatively be made between the pronator teres and flexor carpi radialis muscles (see "Comments" below).

C. Strong retraction between the muscles exposes the joint capsule, which is incised parallel to the muscles. Protect the underlying articular cartilage when making this incision.

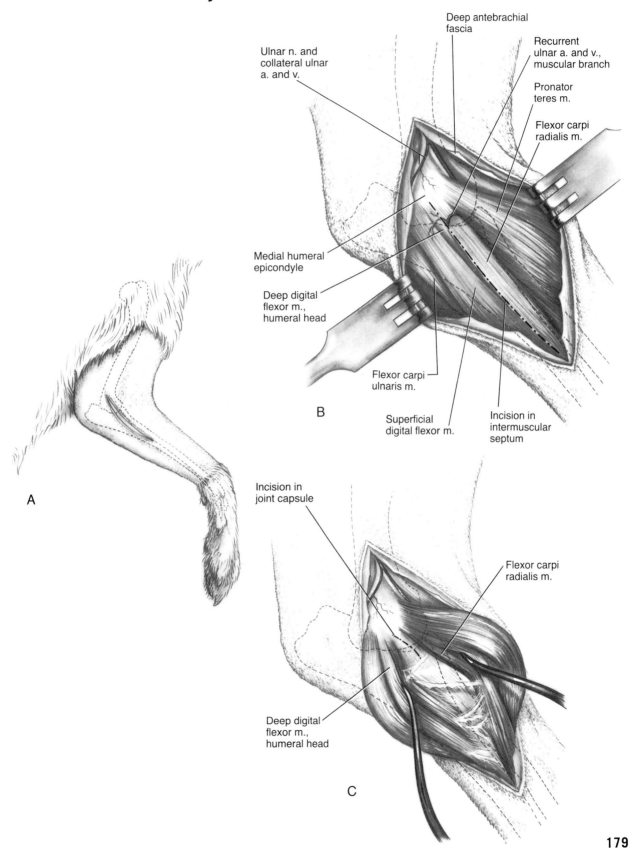

Plate 42

Approach to the Medial Aspect of the Humeral Condyle and the Medial Coronoid Process of the Ulna by an Intermuscular Incision

Deep antebrachial fascia

Ulnar n. and collateral ulnar a. and v.

Recurrent ulnar a. and v., muscular branch

Pronator teres m.

Flexor carpi radialis m.

Medial humeral epicondyle

Deep digital flexor m., humeral head

Flexor carpi ulnaris m.

Superficial digital flexor m.

Incision in intermuscular septum

B

A

Incision in joint capsule

Flexor carpi radialis m.

Deep digital flexor m., humeral head

C

179

Approach to the Medial Aspect of the Humeral Condyle and the Medial Coronoid Process of the Ulna by an Intermuscular Incision *continued*

DESCRIPTION OF THE PROCEDURE *continued*

D. Retraction of the joint capsule exposes the articular surfaces of the humeral condyle and the ulna. Osteochondritis dissecans lesions will be evident on the condyle at this point. Exposure of the medial coronoid process may require extension of the joint capsule incision parallel to the trochlear notch of the ulna, but the incision should not cross the medial collateral ligament.

E. Visualization of the medial coronoid process is facilitated by strong pronation and abduction of the antebrachium to open the joint on the medial side. A sandbag under the drapes or a folded towel on the lateral side of the joint creates a fulcrum for this manuever. A small Hohmann retractor hooked over the coronoid process is also useful.

CLOSURE

Several interrupted sutures are placed in the joint capsule, followed by closure of the intermuscular fascia and the deep fascia. The subcutis and skin are closed in layers.

COMMENTS

This approach as described by Probst and his coworkers placed the intermuscular incision between the pronator teres and flexor carpi radialis muscles. There is little difference in our hands, but there seem to be fewer vascular branches in the intermuscular space used here, and the collateral ligament may be better protected.

Plate 42

Approach to the Medial Aspect of the Humeral Condyle and the Medial Coronoid Process of the Ulna by an Intermuscular Incision *continued*

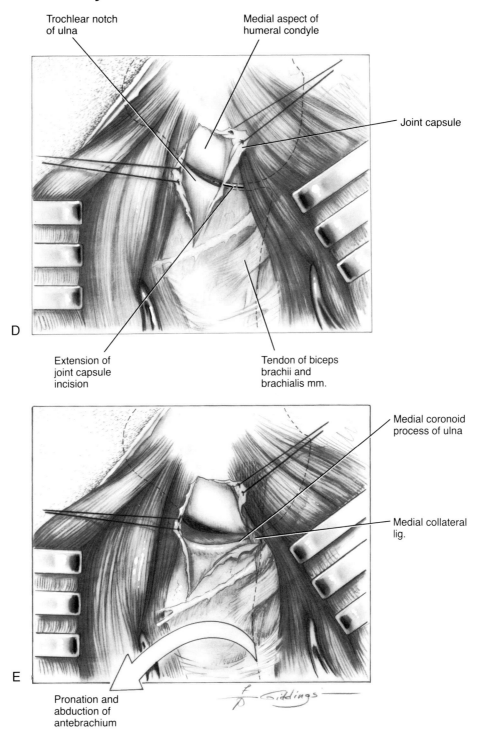

Trochlear notch of ulna

Medial aspect of humeral condyle

Joint capsule

Extension of joint capsule incision

Tendon of biceps brachii and brachialis mm.

D

Medial coronoid process of ulna

Medial collateral lig.

Pronation and abduction of antebrachium

E

Approach to the Medial Aspect of the Humeral Condyle and Medial Coronoid Process of the Ulna By Osteotomy of the Medial Humeral Epicondyle

Based on a Procedure of Stoll[39]

INDICATIONS

1. Osteochondroplasty of the medial aspect of the humeral condyle for osteochondritis dissecans.
2. Excision of fragmented medial coronoid process of the ulna.
3. Open reduction of medial luxation of the head of the radius.

ALTERNATIVE/COMBINATION APPROACH

Plate 42

DESCRIPTION OF THE PROCEDURE

This procedure is initiated as shown in Parts A, B, and C of Plate 41.

A. After incising the deep antebrachial fascia and removing alveolar fat, the epicondylar osteotomy is planned. The osteotomy should include all of the origin of both the pronator teres and flexor carpi radialis muscles. Sharp dissection is necessary to separate fibers of the flexor carpi radialis from the adjacent digital flexor muscles. If the epicondyle is to be reattached with a lag screw (see "Closure" below), a suitable glide and tap hole should be drilled now, just distal to the epicondyle.

B. An osteotome of 10- to 12-mm width works well for a 50- to 70-lb (22- to 32-kg) dog. Incisions 1 and 2 are first made to a depth of approximately 5 mm, and then incision 3 is made parallel to the surface of the condyle, taking care to not include articular cartilage.

Plate 43

Approach to the Medial Aspect of the Humeral Condyle and the Medial Coronoid Process of the Ulna by Osteotomy of the Medial Humeral Epicondyle

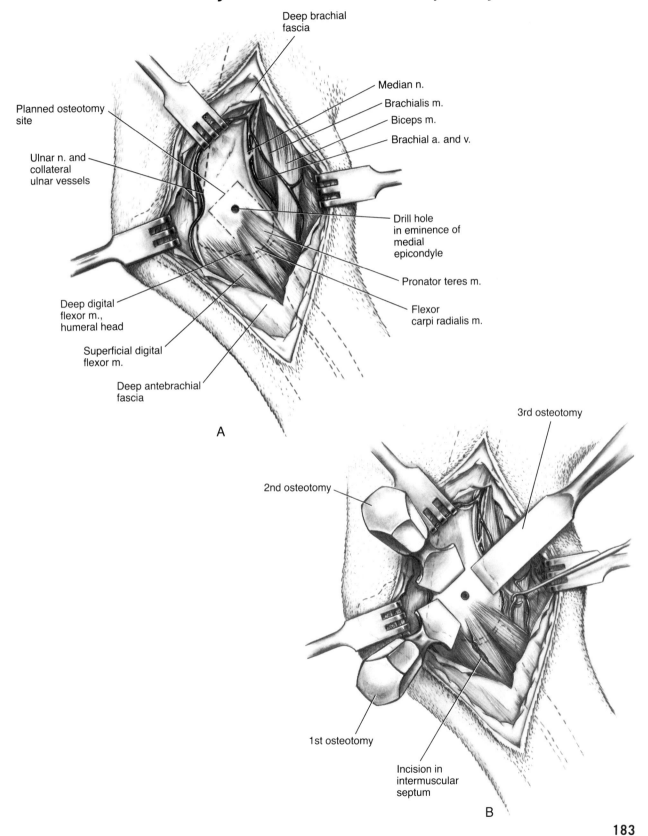

Deep brachial fascia

Median n.

Brachialis m.

Biceps m.

Brachial a. and v.

Planned osteotomy site

Ulnar n. and collateral ulnar vessels

Drill hole in eminence of medial epicondyle

Pronator teres m.

Flexor carpi radialis m.

Deep digital flexor m., humeral head

Superficial digital flexor m.

Deep antebrachial fascia

A

3rd osteotomy

2nd osteotomy

1st osteotomy

Incision in intermuscular septum

B

Approach to the Medial Aspect of the Humeral Condyle and Medial Coronoid Process of the Ulna By Osteotomy of the Medial Humeral Epicondyle *continued*

DESCRIPTION OF THE PROCEDURE *continued*

C. The osteotomized bone with attached muscles and collateral ligaments can be retracted distally after incising the joint capsule. Small Hohmann retractors are useful to expose the condyle and the medial coronoid process. The process is best visualized by abduction and pronation of the forearm.

CLOSURE

Interrupted absorbable sutures are placed in the joint capsule. The osteotomized epicondyle is reattached to its origin by a lag screw or pins and tension-band wire (see Figures 23 and 24). Incisions in the intermuscular septa, deep antebrachial fascia, subcutaneous fascia, and skin are each closed in separate layers.

COMMENTS

The choice of osteotomy or muscle separation is primarily a matter of personal preference. Slightly better exposure is gained here than in the muscle separation approach.

Plate 43

Approach to the Medial Aspect of the Humeral Condyle and the Medial Coronoid Process of the Ulna by Osteotomy of the Medial Humeral Epicondyle *continued*

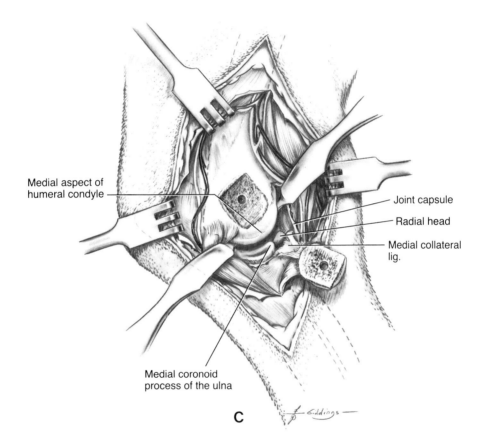

Medial aspect of humeral condyle

Joint capsule

Radial head

Medial collateral lig.

Medial coronoid process of the ulna

C

Approach to the Proximal Shaft and Trochlear Notch of the Ulna

INDICATIONS

1. Open reduction of fractures in the region of the shaft or trochlear notch of the ulna.
2. Open reduction of fracture of ulna and luxation of head of radius (Monteggia fracture).
3. Lengthening and shortening osteotomies of the proximal ulna.

ALTERNATIVE/COMBINATION APPROACHES

Plates 34 through 40, 45, and 46

DESCRIPTION OF THE PROCEDURE

A. The caudal skin incision starts medial to the tuber olecrani and follows the shaft of the ulna distally to the midshaft region. The incision should be 5 to 10 mm medial to the ulnar midline. Subcutaneous and deep antebrachial fascia is incised on the same line.

B. A periosteal incision is made in the origin of the flexor carpi ulnaris muscle on the medial side of the tuber olecrani and shaft of the ulna. A short incision is also necessary in the insertion of the anconeus muscle. This incision continues distally through the fascia between the ulna and the ulnaris lateralis muscle.

C. Subperiosteal elevation and medial retraction of the flexor carpi ulnaris and lateral retraction of the extensor carpi ulnaris muscles expose the ulna. Joint capsule incisions are made as necessary to expose the interior of the joint.

CLOSURE

External fasciae of the flexor and carpi ulnaris and ulnaris lateralis muscles are sutured over the caudal border of the ulna. Deep antebrachial fascia, subcutaneous tissues, and skin are closed in layers.

Plate 44
Approach to the Proximal Shaft and Trochlear Notch of the Ulna

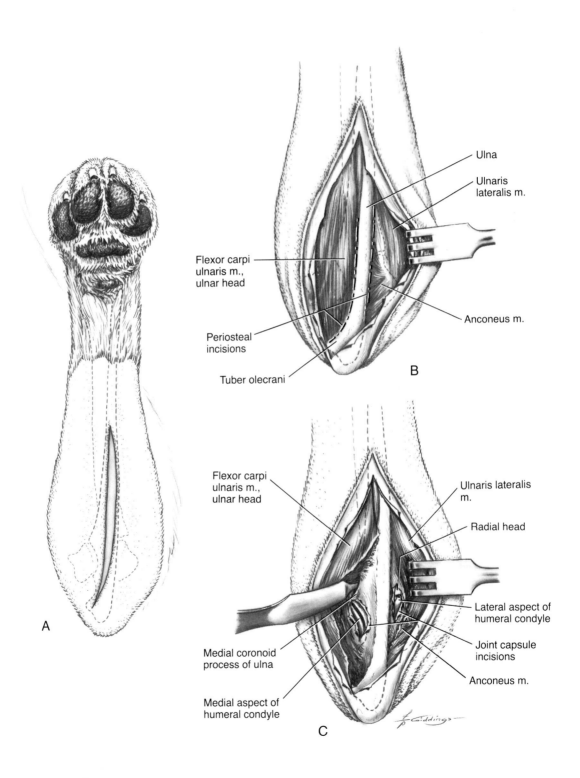

A

B

Ulna

Ulnaris lateralis m.

Flexor carpi ulnaris m., ulnar head

Anconeus m.

Periosteal incisions

Tuber olecrani

C

Flexor carpi ulnaris m., ulnar head

Ulnaris lateralis m.

Radial head

Lateral aspect of humeral condyle

Joint capsule incisions

Anconeus m.

Medial coronoid process of ulna

Medial aspect of humeral condyle

Approach to the Tuber Olecrani

INDICATIONS

1. Open reduction of fractures of the tuber olecrani.
2. Open reduction of fractures of the anconeal process.
3. Excision or fixation of ununited anconeal process.

ALTERNATIVE/COMBINATION APPROACHES

Plates 34 through 40, and 44

DESCRIPTION OF THE PROCEDURE

A. The incision is centered between the lateral humeral epicondyle and the tuber olecrani and curves to follow the humeral condyle proximally and the olecranon distally. Subcutaneous fascia is incised on the same line and elevated with the skin.

B. Brachial fascia is incised parallel to the lateral head of the triceps brachii. A periosteal incision is made in the insertion of the anconeus muscle on the tuber olecrani. This incision continues proximally into the muscle, parallel to its fibers and near the edge of the lateral head of the triceps brachii muscle.

C. Elevation of the anconeus muscle exposes the humeral condyle, anconeal process, and tuber olecrani. If the medial side of the tuber must be exposed to allow for fracture reduction or placement of internal fixation, the flexor carpi ulnaris muscle can be elevated by incising fascia between the muscle and the bone. More proximal elevation of this muscle will require periosteal elevation, as in Plate 44, Part C.

CLOSURE

The intramuscular incision in the anconeus is closed. The insertion of the muscle is sutured to remnants of its insertion or to fascia on the olecranon. The medial fascial incision is closed next, followed by closure of the brachial and subcutaneous fascia and then closure of the skin.

COMMENTS

For excision of an ununited anconeal process, the choice between this approach and the lateral humeroulnar approach shown in Plate 35 is primarily a matter of personal choice.

Plate 45
Approach to the Tuber Olecrani

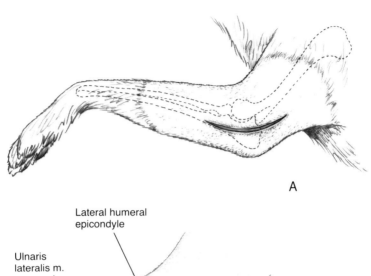

A

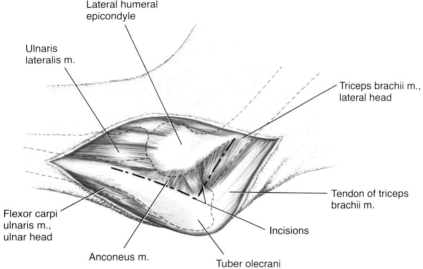

Lateral humeral
epicondyle

Ulnaris
lateralis m.

Triceps brachii m.,
lateral head

Tendon of triceps
brachii m.

Flexor carpi
ulnaris m.,
ulnar head

Anconeus m.

Incisions

Tuber olecrani

B

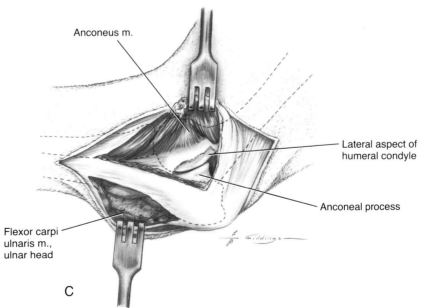

Anconeus m.

Lateral aspect of
humeral condyle

Anconeal process

Flexor carpi
ulnaris m.,
ulnar head

C

Approach to the Distal Shaft and Styloid Process of the Ulna

INDICATIONS

1. Ostectomy or osteotomy of the ulna for treatment of premature distal ulnar physeal closure.
2. Open reduction of fractures.

ALTERNATIVE/COMBINATION APPROACHES

Plates 48, 49, and 50

DESCRIPTION OF THE PROCEDURE

A. The skin incision is made directly over the lateral surface of the bone, from the styloid to about the midshaft.

B. Incision of the subcutaneous tissues allows visualization beneath the antebrachial fascia of the tendon of the ulnaris lateralis muscle directly over, or slightly caudal to, the bone. Likewise, deep to the fascia is the tendon of the lateral digital extensor muscle cranial to the bone. The fascia is incised between the tendons.

C. Retraction of the tendons and fascia exposes the bone. If necessary, part of the origin of the abductor pollicis longus muscle can be elevated from its origin on the cranial border of the ulna and the interosseous ligament (see also Plate 49C and D).

CLOSURE

Closure of the antebrachial fascia is followed by closure of the subcutis and the skin.

Plate 46

Approach to the Distal Shaft and Styloid Process of the Ulna

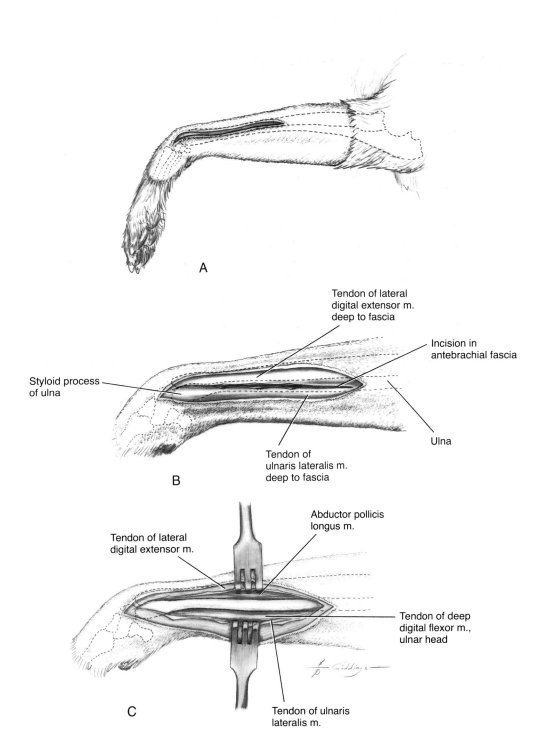

A

Tendon of lateral
digital extensor m.
deep to fascia

Incision in
antebrachial fascia

Styloid process
of ulna

Ulna

Tendon of
ulnaris lateralis m.
deep to fascia

B

Abductor pollicis
longus m.

Tendon of lateral
digital extensor m.

Tendon of deep
digital flexor m.,
ulnar head

Tendon of ulnaris
lateralis m.

C

Approach to the Head and Proximal Metaphysis of the Radius

INDICATIONS

1. Open reduction of fractures.
2. Open reduction of luxation of the radial head.

ALTERNATIVE/COMBINATION APPROACHES

Plates 34, 35, 36, 39, and 40

DESCRIPTION OF THE PROCEDURE

A. The skin is incised from the lateral epicondyle of the humerus on a line following the craniolateral border of the radius to the junction of the proximal and middle one third of the bone.

B. The deep antebrachial fascia is incised on the same line as the skin. The extensor muscles, collateral radial vessels, and a cutaneous branch of the radial nerve will be exposed. An incision is made in the intermuscular septum between the extensor carpi radialis and common digital extensor muscles. This incision starts just distal to the nerve. The vessels must be ligated.

C. Dissection between the extensor muscles allows their retraction and exposure of the supinator muscle. It is important that the deep ramus of the radial nerve be identified and protected throughout the rest of the procedure. Subperiosteal elevation of the supinator's insertion on the radius is begun.

Plate 47

Approach to the Head and Proximal Metaphysis of the Radius

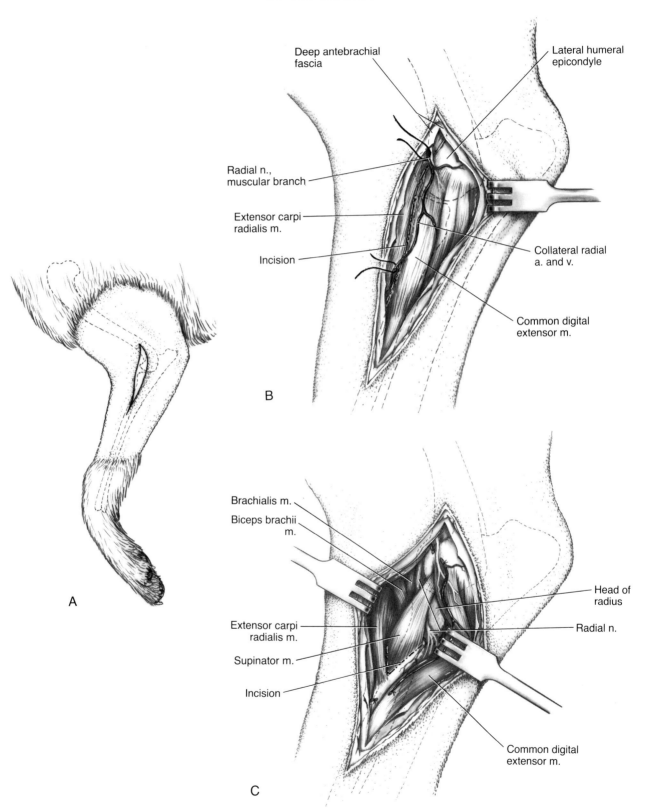

B

Deep antebrachial fascia

Lateral humeral epicondyle

Radial n., muscular branch

Extensor carpi radialis m.

Incision

Collateral radial a. and v.

Common digital extensor m.

A

C

Brachialis m.

Biceps brachii m.

Extensor carpi radialis m.

Supinator m.

Incision

Head of radius

Radial n.

Common digital extensor m.

Approach to the Head and Proximal Metaphysis of the Radius *continued*

DESCRIPTION OF THE PROCEDURE *continued*

D. Elevation of the proximal portion of the muscle insertion must be done carefully to avoid the radial nerve.

E. The radial nerve can be elevated and gently retracted with the supinator to expose the radius.

CLOSURE

There is usually very little of the supinator insertion left on the radius into which sutures can be placed. Sutures are placed in the external fascia of the supinator and attached to any other muscle fascia in the area, such as the pronator teres. The intermuscular septum is closed between the extensor muscles, followed by the deep antebrachial fascia, subcutaneous tissues, and skin.

Plate 47

Approach to the Head and Proximal Metaphysis
of the Radius *continued*

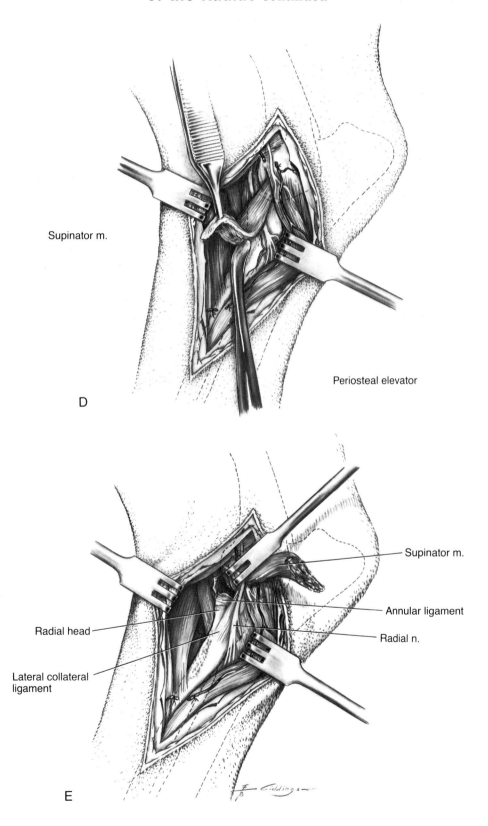

Supinator m.

Periosteal elevator

D

Supinator m.

Annular ligament

Radial n.

Radial head

Lateral collateral
ligament

E

Approach to the Shaft of the Radius Through a Medial Incision

INDICATIONS

1. Open reduction of fractures.
2. Osteotomy of the radius for treatment of radius curvus.

ALTERNATIVE/COMBINATION APPROACHES

Plates 49 and 50

DESCRIPTION OF THE PROCEDURE

A. The skin incision extends from the medial epicondyle of the humerus to the styloid process of the radius. The cephalic vein crosses beneath the distal portion of the incision and is protected during the incision.

B. Subcutaneous fascia is incised on the same line as the skin, and the skin edges are retracted to expose the underlying muscles. The deep antebrachial fascia is incised between the extensor carpi radialis and pronator muscles proximally, with the distal portion of the incision paralleling the extensor muscle. Note the proximity of the brachial artery and vein and median nerve at the proximal end of this incision (shown in more detail in Plate 43, Part A, and below).

Plate 48

Approach to the Shaft of the Radius
Through a Medial Incision

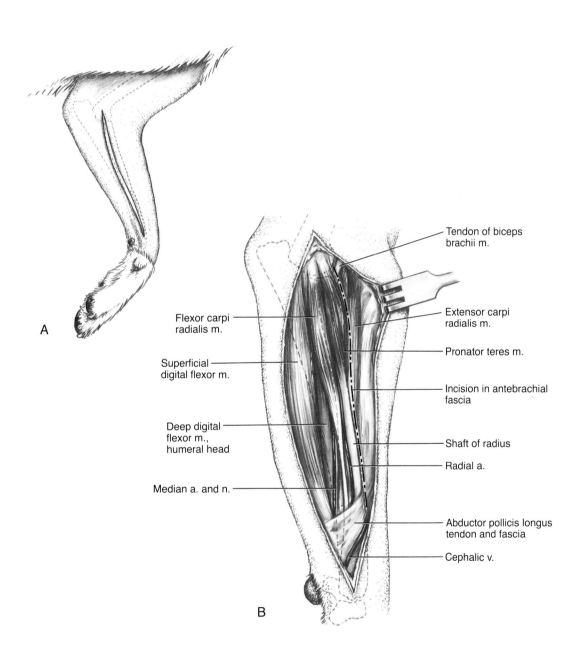

A

Flexor carpi
radialis m.

Superficial
digital flexor m.

Deep digital
flexor m.,
humeral head

Median a. and n.

Tendon of biceps
brachii m.

Extensor carpi
radialis m.

Pronator teres m.

Incision in antebrachial
fascia

Shaft of radius

Radial a.

Abductor pollicis longus
tendon and fascia

Cephalic v.

B

Approach to the Shaft of the Radius Through a Medial Incision *continued*

DESCRIPTION OF THE PROCEDURE *continued*

C. Retraction of the extensor muscles laterally reveals the supinator muscle. If needed for exposure of the proximal radius, the insertions of the pronator and supinator muscles are incised on the radius.

D. Elevation of the pronator and supinator muscles completes the exposure of the proximal portion of the radius. The radial nerve lies deep to the proximal supinator and should be protected (see Plate 47, Part C).

CLOSURE

The pronator and supinator muscles are sutured to their insertions. If insufficient tissue remains at the insertion, these muscles are sutured to adjacent muscles, the pronator quadratus for the supinator and the medial edge of the extensor carpi radialis for the pronator. The deep antebrachial fascia and subcutaneous fascia are closed in separate layers.

COMMENTS

The flexor carpi radialis and deep digital flexor muscles can be elevated caudally for exposure, if necessary, but caution is needed to avoid severing the radial and caudal interosseous arteries that pass between the radius and these muscles. If more exposure is required distally, the skin incision can be curved toward the dorsal surface of the paw. It is then possible to combine this approach with the Approach to the Distal Radius and Carpus Through a Dorsal Incision (Plate 50).

Plate 48

Approach to the Shaft of the Radius
Through a Medial Incision *continued*

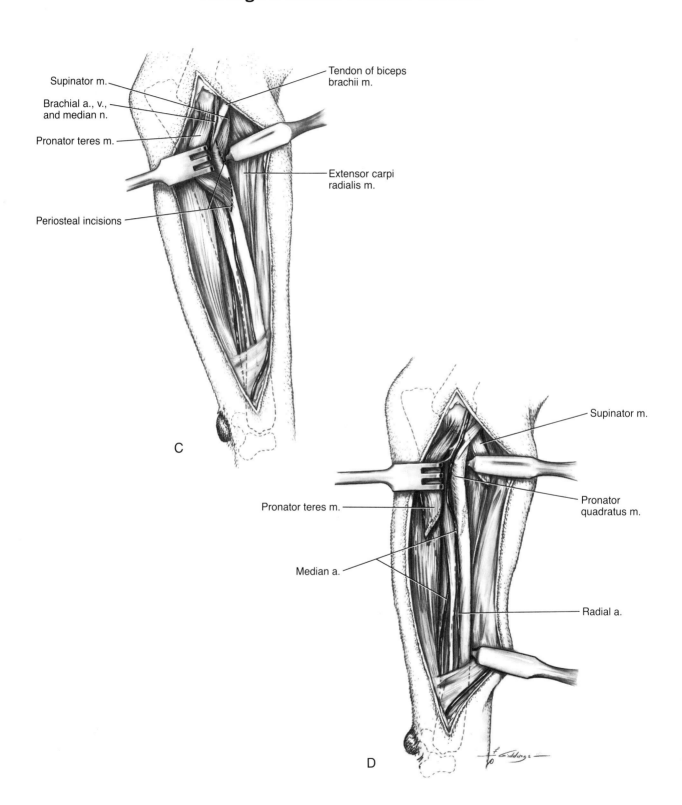

Supinator m.

Brachial a., v., and median n.

Pronator teres m.

Periosteal incisions

Tendon of biceps brachii m.

Extensor carpi radialis m.

C

Supinator m.

Pronator teres m.

Median a.

Pronator quadratus m.

Radial a.

D

Approach to the Shaft of the Radius Through a Lateral Incision

INDICATIONS

1. Open reduction and internal fixation of fractures of the shafts of the radius and ulna.
2. Osteotomy of the radius and ulna.

ALTERNATIVE/COMBINATION APPROACHES

Plates 46, 47, 48, and 50

DESCRIPTION OF THE PROCEDURE

A. The incision is centered over the lateral edge of the radius, starting near the radial head and extending to the distal end of the bone. The subcutaneous fat and superficial antebrachial fascia are incised on the same line.

B. After retracting the skin margins, the shaft of the radius will come into view through the deep antebrachial fascia. This fascia is incised along the cranial border of the common digital extensor muscle to free this muscle for retraction.

Plate 49

Approach to the Shaft of the Radius Through a Lateral Incision

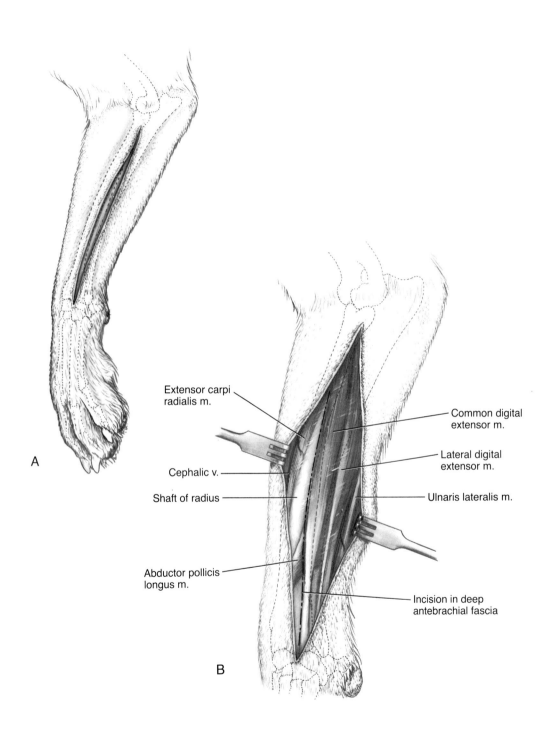

A

Extensor carpi radialis m.

Common digital extensor m.

Cephalic v.

Lateral digital extensor m.

Shaft of radius

Ulnaris lateralis m.

Abductor pollicis longus m.

Incision in deep antebrachial fascia

B

Approach to the Shaft of the Radius Through a Lateral Incision *continued*

DESCRIPTION OF THE PROCEDURE *continued*

C. Caudal retraction of the common and lateral digital extensor muscles exposes most of the shaft of the radius laterally. Better views of the cranial aspect are obtained by medial retraction of the extensor carpi radialis muscle. *If more exposure of the caudolateral aspect of the radius and the ulna is needed,* an incision is made through the abductor pollicis longus muscle near its origin on the ulna and parallel to the muscle extensor pollicis longus et indicis proprius.

D. Retraction of the extensor muscles provides complete exposure of the shafts of the radius and ulna.

CLOSURE

The abductor pollicis longus muscle is either reattached to its origin on the ulna or sutured to the cranial border of the extensor pollicis muscle. The deep antebrachial fascia is closed separately from the superficial fascia/subcutaneous fat layer. The skin is closed routinely.

COMMENTS

In the case of fractures, the choice between this lateral approach and the medial approach (see Plate 48) is often simply personal preference. However, if there is a need to reduce and apply fixation to the ulna in support of the radial fixation, this approach is superior to the medial approach. Soft tissue injuries may dictate which side to choose. When doing a distal radial and ulnar osteotomy, this approach is easily combined with the lateral approach to the ulna (see Plate 46) to allow both osteotomies through a single skin incision.

Plate 49

Approach to the Shaft of the Radius Through a Lateral Incision *continued*

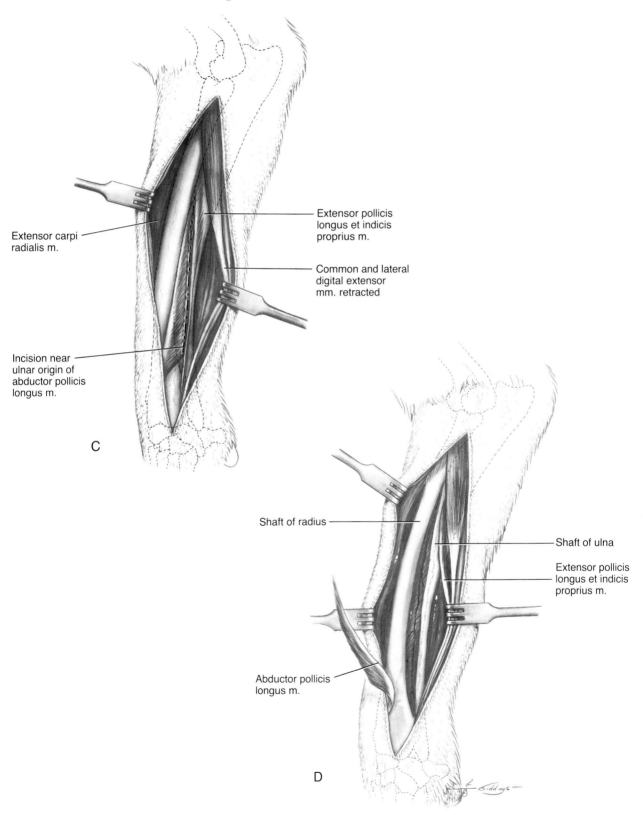

Extensor carpi radialis m.

Extensor pollicis longus et indicis proprius m.

Common and lateral digital extensor mm. retracted

Incision near ulnar origin of abductor pollicis longus m.

C

Shaft of radius

Shaft of ulna

Extensor pollicis longus et indicis proprius m.

Abductor pollicis longus m.

D

Approach to the Distal Radius and Carpus Through a Dorsal Incision

Based on a Procedure of Hurov et al.[20]

INDICATIONS

1. Open reduction of fractures of the distal radius or carpal bones.
2. Open reduction of luxations of the joint.
3. Arthrodesis of the carpus.

DESCRIPTION OF THE PROCEDURE

A. An Esmarch bandage and tourniquet can be used below the elbow. The skin incision is made on the mid-dorsal surface of the joint and extends from the juncture of the cephalic and accessory cephalic veins to the middle of the metacarpus. The incision is lateral to the accessory cephalic vein and curves laterally at its distal end to follow the vein.

Subcutaneous fascia is likewise incised just lateral to the vein, enough fascia being left on the vein to allow the placing of sutures in this tissue during closure. The vein and fascia are undermined and retracted medially with the skin.

B. The deep antebrachial fascia is incised midway between the tendon of the extensor carpi radialis and the tendon of the common digital extensor. The usual limits of incision are the abductor pollicis longus muscle proximally and the proximal metacarpal bones distally (see "Comments" below). The incision is then deepened to penetrate the periosteum on the distal end of the radius.

C. The periosteum is elevated medially and laterally to allow the retraction of the tendons without disturbing their sheaths. The fat pad attached to the extensor carpi radialis tendon may be trimmed, if necessary, to allow visualization of the joint cavity. The styloid process of the ulna may be exposed by continued lateral elevation of the periosteum and retraction of the lateral digital extensor tendon. Synovial incisions are made at the desired joints.

D. Because the synovium is adherent to the dorsal surfaces of individual carpal bones, the joint capsule must be incised around each bone in order to expose it. Exposure of the various joint spaces is enhanced by flexion of the carpus.

CLOSURE

There is usually little synovium available for closure. Simply close the deep and superficial fascial layers over the tendons, before closing the skin.

COMMENTS

The exposure can be increased proximally by incising the abductor pollicis muscle; this will usually be necessary for bone plate application. The muscle is sutured with mattress sutures.

Plate 50

Approach to the Distal Radius and Carpus
Through a Dorsal Incision

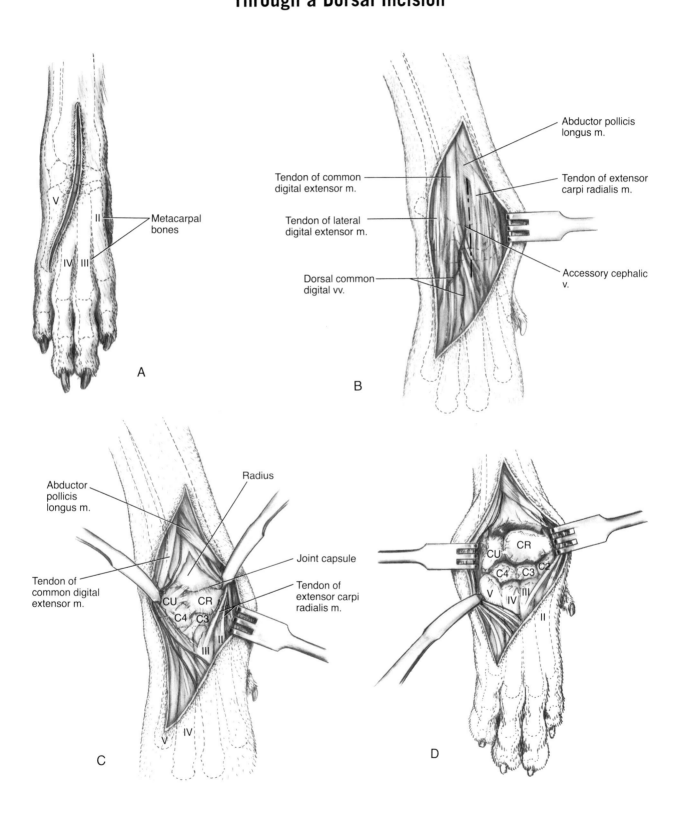

A

V

II

IV III

Metacarpal bones

B

Tendon of common digital extensor m.

Tendon of lateral digital extensor m.

Dorsal common digital vv.

Abductor pollicis longus m.

Tendon of extensor carpi radialis m.

Accessory cephalic v.

C

Abductor pollicis longus m.

Radius

Tendon of common digital extensor m.

Joint capsule

Tendon of extensor carpi radialis m.

CU   CR

C4   C3

II

III

V   IV

D

CR

CU   C2

C4   C3

V   III

IV

II

Approach to the Distal Radius and Carpus Through a Palmaromedial Incision

INDICATIONS

1. Panarthrodesis of carpus with palmar bone plate.
2. Fixation of caudal fractures of distal radius.
3. Removal of bone fragments from carpal joints.

ALTERNATIVE/COMBINATION APPROACHES

Plates 50 and 52

DESCRIPTION OF THE PROCEDURE

A. The longitudinal skin incision is equidistant between the radial styloid process and the carpal pad. A longer incision is needed for palmar bone plating.

B. The cephalic vein is double ligated and divided. An incision is made in the midportion of the flexor retinacular fascia and lengthened proximally into the antebrachial fascia as needed.

C. Upon retracting the retinacular fascia, the tendons of the flexor carpi radialis and the digital flexor muscles, as well as the median artery and nerve, will be visible. Branches of the vessels and nerves to the first digit are isolated and the vessels ligated. The flexor tendon can be divided, or simply retracted, depending on the exposure required.

   N.B. Due to the anatomic complexity of this region, considerable license has been taken with Parts D and E. Omitted for clarity are the lumbricales, interosseus, adductor digiti secundi, and adductor/flexor pollicis muscles. Also deleted are the palmar carpal fibrocartilage and the palmar ligamentous structure. These tissues are incised and retracted as necessary to achieve the exposure depicted here.

Plate 51

Approach to the Distal Radius and Carpus
Through a Palmaromedial Incision

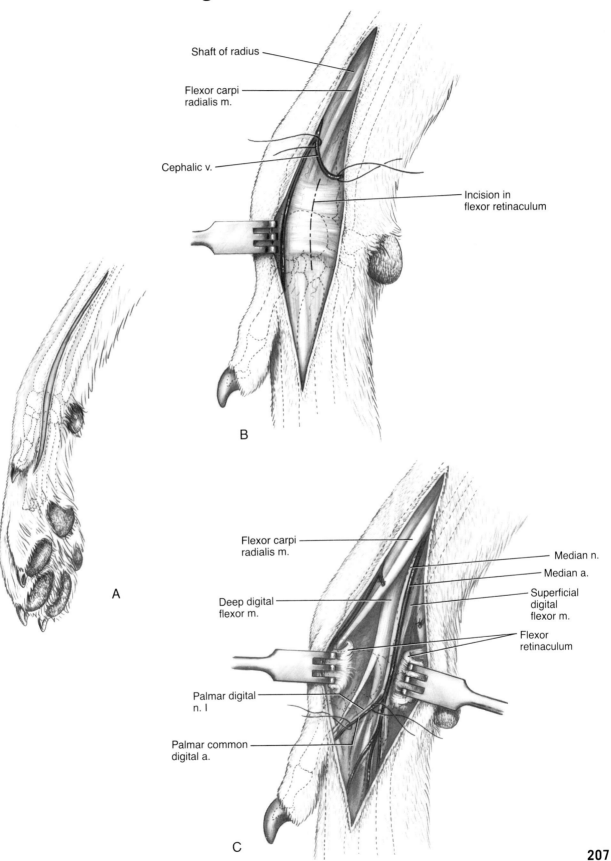

Shaft of radius

Flexor carpi
radialis m.

Cephalic v.

Incision in
flexor retinaculum

B

A

Flexor carpi
radialis m.

Median n.

Median a.

Deep digital
flexor m.

Superficial
digital
flexor m.

Flexor
retinaculum

Palmar digital
n. I

Palmar common
digital a.

C

207

Approach to the Distal Radius and Carpus Through a Palmaromedial Incision *continued*

DESCRIPTION OF THE PROCEDURE *continued*

D. Retraction of the digital flexor tendons exposes the palmar carpal region superficially. The entire region will be covered by a combination of joint capsule, ligaments, and palmar carpal fibrocartilage. The desired joint spaces are identified by probing with a hypodermic needle. Incisions in the appropriate spaces are then made. Be aware of the deep palmar arch and palmar metacarpal arteries as these incisions are made.

E. Incisions in the joint capsules of the various joints are extended as needed.

CLOSURE

Unless an arthrodesis has been done, the joint capsule/ligament/fibrocartilage incisions are closed with interrupted sutures of nonabsorbable or polydioxanone/polyglyconate materials. The flexor retinaculum and deep antebrachial fascia are similarly closed. There is usually not enough subcutaneous tissue to warrant suturing.

COMMENTS

External support by cast or splint is needed for several weeks to allow healing of the palmar carpal structures.

Plate 51

Approach to the Distal Radius and Carpus
Through a Palmaromedial Incision *continued*

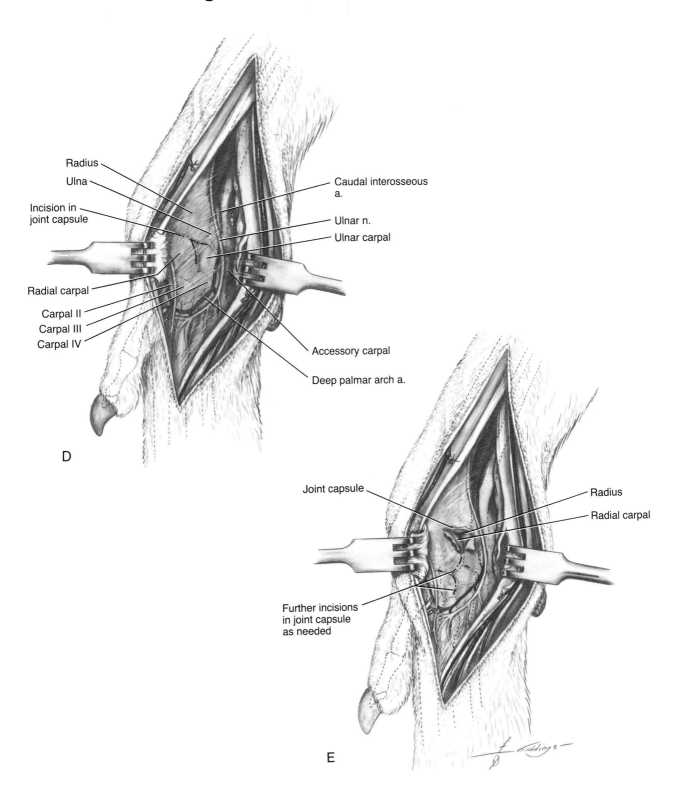

Radius

Ulna

Incision in
joint capsule

Caudal interosseous
a.

Ulnar n.

Ulnar carpal

Radial carpal

Carpal II

Carpal III

Carpal IV

Accessory carpal

Deep palmar arch a.

D

Joint capsule

Radius

Radial carpal

Further incisions
in joint capsule
as needed

E

Approach to the Accessory Carpal Bone and Palmarolateral Carpal Joints

INDICATIONS

1. Internal fixation of fractures of the accessory carpal bone.
2. Internal fixation of fractures of the palmar process of the ulnar carpal bone.
3. Ligamentous reconstructive procedures.

DESCRIPTION OF THE PROCEDURE

A. The skin incision is made from the caudomedial border of the distal ulna, curving laterally around the accessory carpal bone and ending distally over the palmar side of the fifth metacarpal bone. Subcutaneous fascia is incised on the same line.

B. Deep fascia intimately connects the carpal pad to the free end of the accessory carpal bone. This fascia is partially dissected to allow medial retraction of the skin and pad. Extending laterally from the free end of the accessory carpal and inserting on the tendon of the ulnaris lateralis tendon is the lateral flexor retinaculum, which is incised near the accessory carpal bone. This will allow sharp dissection to free the abductor digiti quinti muscle from its origin on the accessory carpal bone. The muscle is freed from between the two accessory metacarpal ligaments and reflected distally (see "Comments" below).

C. Retraction of the accessory metacarpal ligaments will reveal the distomedial surface of the accessory carpal bone, the most common site of fractures.

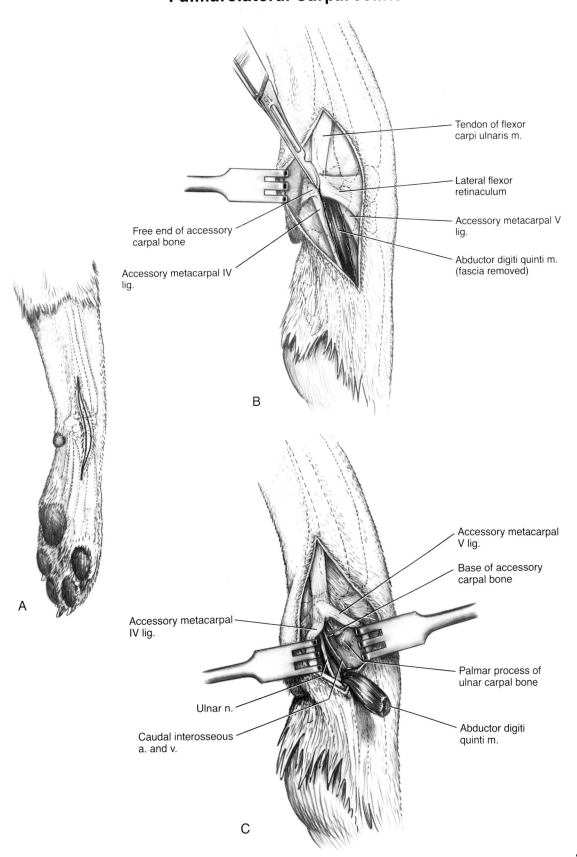

Plate 52

Approach to the Accessory Carpal Bone and Palmarolateral Carpal Joints

Tendon of flexor carpi ulnaris m.

Lateral flexor retinaculum

Accessory metacarpal V lig.

Abductor digiti quinti m. (fascia removed)

Free end of accessory carpal bone

Accessory metacarpal IV lig.

B

Accessory metacarpal V lig.

Base of accessory carpal bone

Accessory metacarpal IV lig.

Palmar process of ulnar carpal bone

Ulnar n.

Caudal interosseous a. and v.

Abductor digiti quinti m.

A

C

211

Approach to the Accessory Carpal Bone and Palmarolateral Carpal Joints *continued*

DESCRIPTION OF THE PROCEDURE *continued*

D, E. To open the palmarolateral aspect of the antebrachiocarpal joint, the accessory carpal bone is retracted medially to help identify the joint space along its lateral border. This joint capsule is incised from the ulnar styloid process around the lateral side of the accessory carpal and onto the palmar process of the ulnar carpal bone. Try to leave some capsule tissue on the accessory carpal to allow for suturing. Strong medial and distal retraction of the free end of the accessory carpal bone will expose most of the articular surface and allow removal of small bone fragments.

CLOSURE

The joint capsule incision is closed with interrupted-pattern 3/0 or 4/0 nonabsorbable or polydioxanone/polyglyconate sutures. The abductor digiti quinti muscle is reattached to the accessory metacarpal ligaments; the flexor retinaculum is likewise closed with interrupted sutures, followed by closure of the skin.

COMMENTS

The abductor digiti quinti muscle does not need to be detached to make the joint capsule incision. The only purpose of reflecting the muscle is to allow inspection of the distomedial surface of the accessory carpal bone.

Plate 52

Approach to the Accessory Carpal Bone and Palmarolateral Carpal Joints *continued*

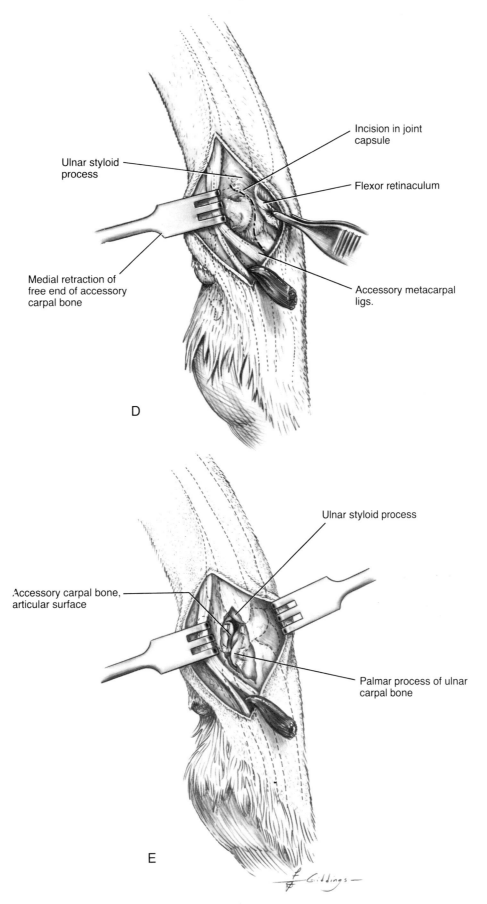

Ulnar styloid process

Incision in joint capsule

Flexor retinaculum

Medial retraction of free end of accessory carpal bone

Accessory metacarpal ligs.

D

Ulnar styloid process

Accessory carpal bone, articular surface

Palmar process of ulnar carpal bone

E

Approaches to the Metacarpal Bones

INDICATION

Open reduction of fractures.

DESCRIPTION OF THE PROCEDURE

A. The anatomy shown here is considerably simplified compared to that in a live animal. Only the important structures are shown; other elements, such as small tendons and blood vessels, have been omitted. In an average-sized dog, these vestigial structures are so small that their identification and preservation are not practical during surgery.

B, C, D. The incisional technique varies according to the bone or bones to be exposed. A single bone is approached by an incision directly over the bone, and two adjoining bones by an incision between them. If more than two bones need be exposed, two parallel longitudinal incisions (Part B) or a single curved incision (Part C) can be used. The curved incision commences at the proximal end of metacarpal II, runs laterally to the midshaft of metacarpal V, and then curves medially again to end over the distal end of metacarpal II. The crescent-shaped skin flap can be elevated and retracted to expose a large part of all four bones. Another alternative is two parallel incisions connected to form an "H" (Part D).

To expose metacarpals II and III, the deep fascia is incised over bone II, and the vessels and tendons are then undermined and retracted laterally. Deep fascia is incised over bone V to expose bones IV and V. Tendons and vessels are again undermined and retracted medially. Exposure of bone IV sometimes requires an incision between tendons, followed by sufficient dissection of the tendons from the surrounding fascia to allow their separation and retraction.

CLOSURE

Deep fascia is closed to ensure that tendons and vessels are securely held in their proper positions.

COMMENTS

A deep layer of small metacarpal blood vessels is found on and between the bones. These vessels are too small to avoid in most animals, and the resulting hemorrhage must be controlled by tamponade. Use of an Esmarch bandage and a tourniquet is very helpful. Do not leave the tourniquet in place for more than 1½ hours, and apply a snug bandange for 72 hours postoperatively to control oozing hemorrhage at the operative site.

Plate 53

Approaches to the Metacarpal Bones

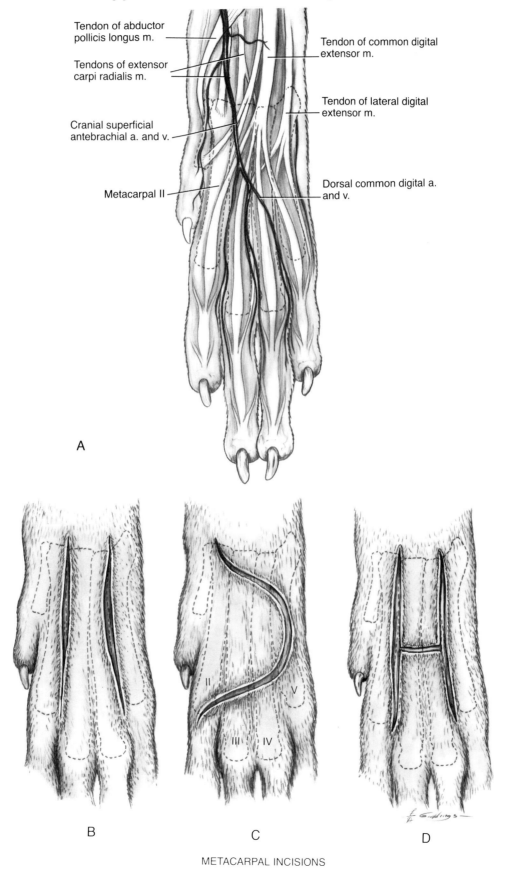

Tendon of abductor pollicis longus m.

Tendons of extensor carpi radialis m.

Cranial superficial antebrachial a. and v.

Metacarpal II

Tendon of common digital extensor m.

Tendon of lateral digital extensor m.

Dorsal common digital a. and v.

A

B

C

D

METACARPAL INCISIONS

215

Approach to the Proximal Sesamoid Bones

INDICATION

Excision of fractured sesamoid bones.

DESCRIPTION OF THE PROCEDURE

A. The most commonly fractured sesamoid bones, in both the fore and hind paws, are those of metacarpal or metatarsal II and V. The skin incision curves around the metacarpal or metatarsal pad. A medial incision can be used for metacarpals (metatarsals) II and III, and a lateral incision for IV and V.

B. After reflection of the skin, the sesamoid bones are palpated at the metacarpophalangeal (metatarsophalangeal) joint. A vertical incision is made in the manica flexoria and the sheath of the superficial digital flexor tendon directly over the sesamoids.

C. Retraction of the manica flexoria and sheath of the superficial digital flexor tendon reveals the paired sesamoid bones under the digital flexor tendons. The tendons can be retracted in either direction to expose the sesamoid bones. If the bone is fractured at about the midportion, the entire bone is removed. If fractured toward the end of the bone, only the smaller fragment is removed. Removal consists of sharply dissecting away the intersesmoidean, lateral, medial, and cruciate ligaments of the sesamoid bones.

CLOSURE

Interrupted sutures of 3/0 to 4/0 nonabsorbable or polydioxanone acid material are placed in the manica flexoria superficial digital flexor tendon sheath incision. The skin is closed next, it being unnecessary to close the subcutaneous tissue.

COMMENT

A padded bandage should be worn for 10 days.

Plate 54

Approach to the Proximal Sesamoid Bones

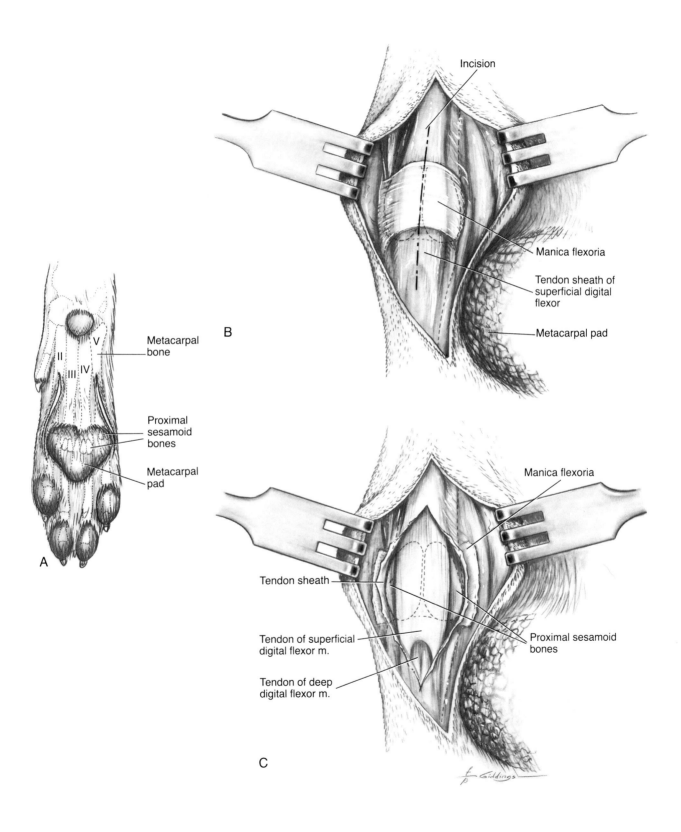

A

Metacarpal bone

Proximal sesamoid bones

Metacarpal pad

B

Incision

Manica flexoria

Tendon sheath of superficial digital flexor

Metacarpal pad

C

Manica flexoria

Tendon sheath

Proximal sesamoid bones

Tendon of superficial digital flexor m.

Tendon of deep digital flexor m.

Approaches to the Phalanges and Interphalangeal Joints

INDICATIONS

1. Open reduction of fractures of phalanges.
2. Open reduction of luxations of metatarso- or metacarpophalangeal and interphalangeal joints.

DESCRIPTION OF THE PROCEDURE

A. An Esmarch bandage and tourniquet can be used on the lower limb. The skin incision starts at the distal end of the appropriate metacarpal bone, proceeds distally over the dorsal surface of the phalanges, and ends over the distal phalanx. If the distal interphalangeal joint is to be exposed, a transverse incision can be made at the distal end of the vertical incision to form a "T."

B. Sharp dissection is used to reflect skin flaps away from underlying bones and tendons.

CLOSURE

Due to the scarcity of subcutaneous tissues, the skin is often the only layer to be closed.

COMMENTS

A snug, padded bandage should be worn for 10 days, unless the foot is splinted.

Plate 55

Approaches to the Phalanges and Interphalangeal Joints

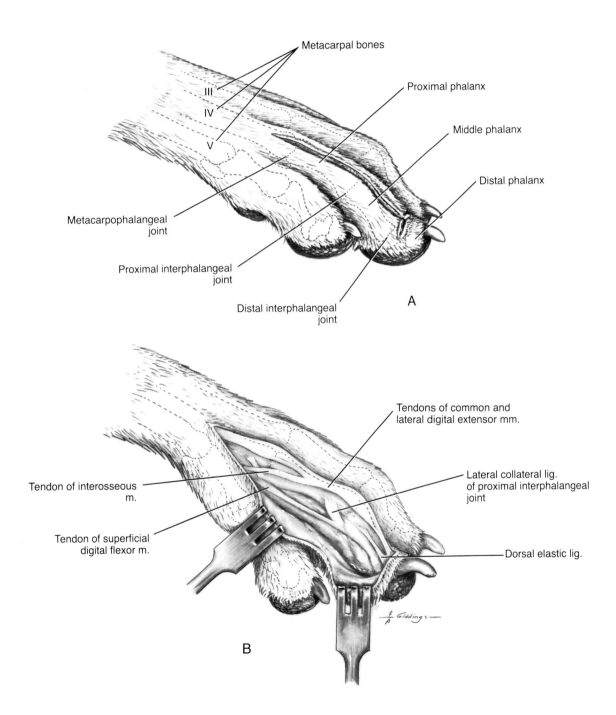

Metacarpal bones

Proximal phalanx

Middle phalanx

Distal phalanx

III

IV

V

Metacarpophalangeal joint

Proximal interphalangeal joint

Distal interphalangeal joint

A

Tendons of common and lateral digital extensor mm.

Lateral collateral lig. of proximal interphalangeal joint

Tendon of interosseous m.

Tendon of superficial digital flexor m.

Dorsal elastic lig.

B

The Pelvis and Hip Joint

- Approach to the Wing of the Ilium and Dorsal Aspect of the Sacrum

- Approach to the Ilium Through a Lateral Incision

- Approach to the Ventral Aspect of the Sacrum

- Approach to the Craniodorsal Aspect of the Hip Joint Through a Craniolateral Incision

- Approach to the Dorsal Aspect of the Hip Joint Through an Intergluteal Incision

- Approach to the Craniodorsal and Caudodorsal Aspects of the Hip Joint by Osteotomy of the Greater Trochanter

- Approach to the Craniodorsal and Caudodorsal Aspects of the Hip Joint by Tenotomy of the Gluteal Muscles

- Approach to the Caudal Aspect of the Hip Joint and Body of the Ischium

- Approach to the Os Coxae

- Approach to the Ventral Aspect of the Hip Joint or the Ramus of the Pubis

- Approach to the Pubis and Pelvic Symphysis

- Approach to the Ischium

Approach to the Wing of the Ilium and Dorsal Aspect of the Sacrum

Based on a Procedure of Alexander, Archibald and Cawley[2]

INDICATIONS

1. Open reduction of sacroiliac luxations.
2. Open reduction of fractures of the wing of the ilium.
3. Collection of autogenous cancellous bone chips for grafting.

ALTERNATIVE/COMBINATION APPROACHES

Plates 20 and 58

DESCRIPTION OF THE PROCEDURE

A. The animal can be positioned in either lateral (illustrated) or sternal recumbency. The skin incision starts cranially over the cranial dorsal iliac spine and continues caudally parallel to the midline to near the hip joint. Subcutaneous tissues and gluteal fascia and fat are incised on the same line to expose the cranial and caudal dorsal iliac spines.

B. If only the lateral (gluteal) surface of the wing of the ilium need be exposed, as for fractures or cancellous bone collection, an incision is made in the periosteal origin of the middle gluteal muscle on the lateral edge of the ilium near the cranial dorsal iliac spine and ending beyond the caudal dorsal spine. If the sacrum must also be exposed, a second incision is made in the periosteal origin of the sacrospinalis muscle, at the medial edge of the ilium. These incisions merge as they continue caudally, and it will be necessary to incise through some fibers of the superficial gluteal muscle in this area.

C. The middle gluteal muscle is elevated subperiosteally in young animals, or simply scraped from its origin on the ilium in older animals. The elevation continues caudally to the caudal dorsal iliac spine. Continuing further caudal dissection will result in severance of the cranial gluteal artery, vein, and nerve (exposure of the shaft of the ilium is better done by the Approach to the Ilium Through a Lateral Incision, Plate 57). Similar elevation of the sacrospinalis muscle on the medial side of the ilium gives limited exposure of the dorsal surface of the sacrum. Muscular elevation on the sacrum should be confined to the area lateral to the intermediate crests to avoid damage to dorsal nerve roots emerging through the dorsal foramina of the sacrum.

CLOSURE

Superficial fascia of the sacrospinalis and middle gluteal muscles is joined by a row of sutures crossing the wing of the ilium. Caudal to this, the fascia of the superficial gluteal muscle is sutured. This is followed by layer closure of the gluteal fascia, the gluteal fat and subcutaneous fascia, and the skin.

Plate 56

Approach to the Wing of the Ilium and Dorsal Aspect of the Sacrum

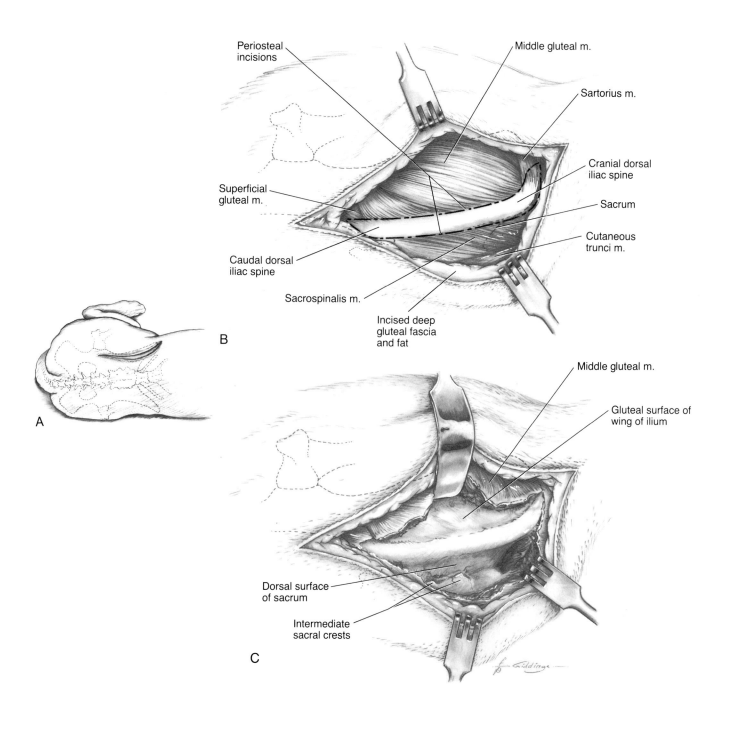

B

Periosteal incisions

Middle gluteal m.

Sartorius m.

Cranial dorsal iliac spine

Sacrum

Cutaneous trunci m.

Superficial gluteal m.

Caudal dorsal iliac spine

Sacrospinalis m.

Incised deep gluteal fascia and fat

A

C

Middle gluteal m.

Gluteal surface of wing of ilium

Dorsal surface of sacrum

Intermediate sacral crests

Approach to the Ilium Through a Lateral Incision

Based on a Procedure of Hohn and Janes[18]

INDICATIONS

1. Open reduction of fractures of the wing and shaft of the ilium.
2. Combined with dorsal approaches to the hip, for exposure of the os coxae.

ALTERNATIVE/COMBINATION APPROACHES

Plates 59, 61, 62, and 64

DESCRIPTION OF THE PROCEDURE

A. The skin incision extends from the center of the iliac crest and ends just caudal and distal to the greater trochanter.

B. Subcutaneous tissues, gluteal fat, and superficial fascia are incised and elevated with the skin. Incision of the deep gluteal fascia on the same line as the skin allows incision of the intermuscular septum between the tensor fasciae latae and middle gluteal muscles. This incision extends from the ventral iliac spine to the cranial border of the biceps femoris muscle. Fascia is also incised along the cranial border of the biceps femoris muscle to create a T-shaped fascial incision.

C, D. Retraction of the middle gluteal muscle exposes the deep gluteal muscle and a portion of the iliac shaft. An incision is made in the origin of the middle gluteal muscle on the ilium, starting at the caudal ventral iliac spine and continuing cranially and dorsally as needed. Some sharp dissection may be needed between the middle gluteal and sartorius muscles. The iliolumbar vessels are ligated at the ventral edge of the ilium. An incision is started in the origin of the deep gluteal muscle, to allow caudal retraction of the muscle.

Plate 57

Approach to the Ilium Through a Lateral Incision *continued*

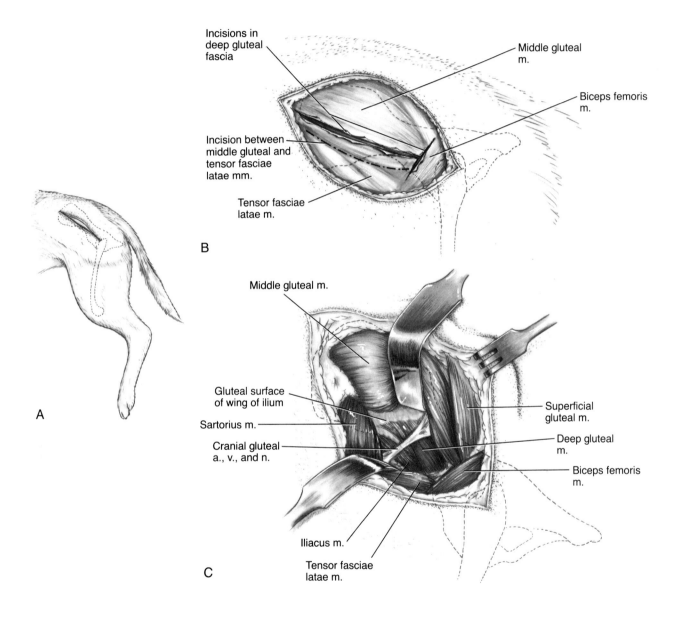

B

Incisions in deep gluteal fascia

Middle gluteal m.

Biceps femoris m.

Incision between middle gluteal and tensor fasciae latae mm.

Tensor fasciae latae m.

A

C

Middle gluteal m.

Gluteal surface of wing of ilium

Sartorius m.

Cranial gluteal a., v., and n.

Superficial gluteal m.

Deep gluteal m.

Biceps femoris m.

Iliacus m.

Tensor fasciae latae m.

Approach to the Ilium Through a Lateral Incision *continued*

DESCRIPTION OF THE PROCEDURE *continued*

E. Subperiosteal elevation of the gluteal muscles exposes the crest, wing, and shaft of the ilium.

Maximal exposure of the shaft of the ilium, cranial to the acetabulum, may necessitate sacrificing branches of the cranial gluteal artery, vein, and nerve that supply the tensor fasciae latae muscle. Elevation of the iliacus muscle along the ventral border of the iliac shaft usually results in severing a nutrient artery on the ventral aspect of the shaft. The severed artery must then be cauterized or plugged with bone wax.

CLOSURE

Sutures are placed between fasciae of the middle gluteal muscle and the sartorius muscle. This suture line continues caudally between middle gluteal and tensor fasciae latae muscles. Deep gluteal fat and fascia, subcutaneous tissues, and skin are approximated in layers.

COMMENTS

Consideration must be given to the sciatic nerve when retracting muscle or using bone holding forceps on the ilium. The nerve lies close to the dorsomedial aspect of the iliac shaft. With care in retracting, the cranial gluteal vessels and nerve can usually be preserved.

Plate 57

Approach to the Ilium Through a Lateral Incision

continued

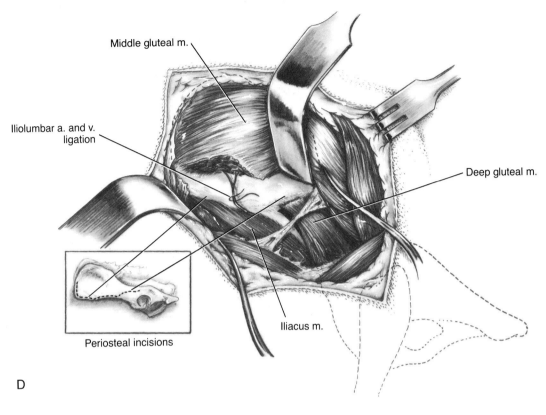

Middle gluteal m.

Iliolumbar a. and v. ligation

Deep gluteal m.

Iliacus m.

Periosteal incisions

D

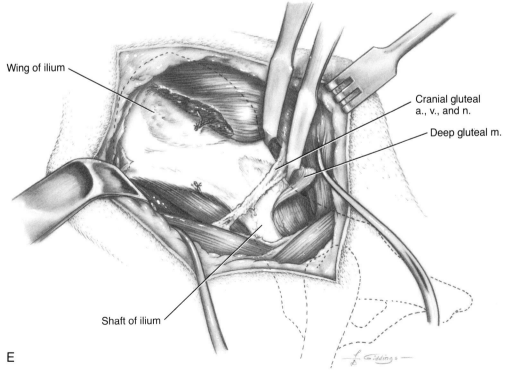

Wing of ilium

Cranial gluteal a., v., and n.

Deep gluteal m.

Shaft of ilium

E

Approach to the Ventral Aspect of the Sacrum

Based on a Procedure of Montavon, Boudrieau, and Hohn[22]

INDICATION

Internal fixation of sacroiliac joint fracture–luxation.

ALTERNATIVE/COMBINATION APPROACHES

Plates 56 and 57

DESCRIPTION OF THE PROCEDURE

This approach is an extension of the Approach to the Ilium Through a Lateral Incision (Plate 57), and parts A–C should be completed as shown. Part D is modified to eliminate elevation of the deep gluteal muscle.

A. The iliacus muscle is incised at its origin along the ventromedial border of the ilium and is subperiosteally elevated sufficiently to allow insertion of a finger into the pelvic canal. The nutrient artery of the ilium may be disrupted during this elevation and is best controlled by bone wax.

B. The body of the sacrum is palpable now; in the case of a sacroiliac luxation, the whole ilial body and wing are mobile enough that the region of the synchondrosis can be palpated on the medial side of the ilium, and the smooth articular surface can be felt on the sacrum.

CLOSURE

Sutures are placed between the fasciae of the middle gluteal and sartorius muscles, and this suture line is continued caudally between the middle gluteal and tensor fasciae latae muscles. Deep gluteal fascia and fat, subcutis, and skin are closed in layers.

COMMENTS

Direct visualization of the sacroiliac joint is useful when fractures are present. This can be accomplished by extending the muscle elevation craniodorsally around the iliac crest to join with the Approach to the Wing of the Ilium and Dorsal Aspect of the Sacrum (Plate 56).

Plate 58

Approach to the Ventral Aspect of the Sacrum

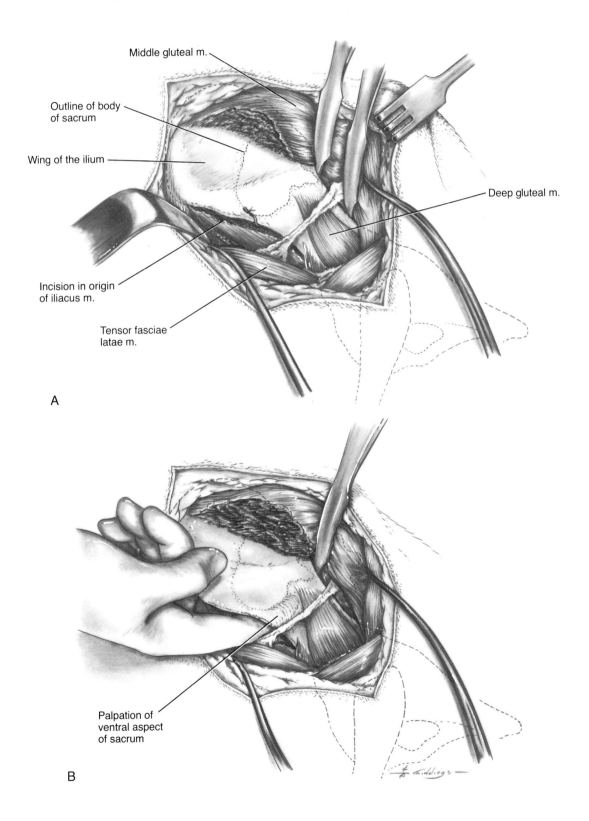

Middle gluteal m.

Outline of body of sacrum

Wing of the ilium

Deep gluteal m.

Incision in origin of iliacus m.

Tensor fasciae latae m.

A

Palpation of ventral aspect of sacrum

B

Approach to the Craniodorsal Aspect of the Hip Joint Through a Craniolateral Incision

Based on Procedures of Archibald et al.[3] and Brown and Rosen[6]

INDICATIONS

1. Femoral head and neck resection.
2. Open reduction of fractures of the femoral head and neck.
3. Open reduction of coxofemoral luxations.
4. Installation of total hip prosthesis.

ALTERNATIVE/COMBINATION APPROACHES

Plates 60, 61, and 62

DESCRIPTION OF THE PROCEDURE

A. The skin incision is centered at the level of the greater trochanter and lies over the cranial border of the shaft of the femur. Distally, it extends one third to one half the length of the femur; proximally, it curves slightly cranially to end just short of the dorsal midline.

B. The skin margins are undermined and retracted. An incision is made through the superficial leaf of the fascia lata, along the cranial border of the biceps femoris muscle.

C. The biceps femoris muscle is retracted caudally to allow incision in the deep leaf of the fascia lata to free the insertion of the tensor fasciae latae muscle. The incision continues proximally through intermuscular septum between the cranial border of the superficial gluteal muscle and the tensor fasciae latae muscle.

Plate 59

Approach to the Craniodorsal Aspect of the Hip Joint Through a Craniolateral Incision

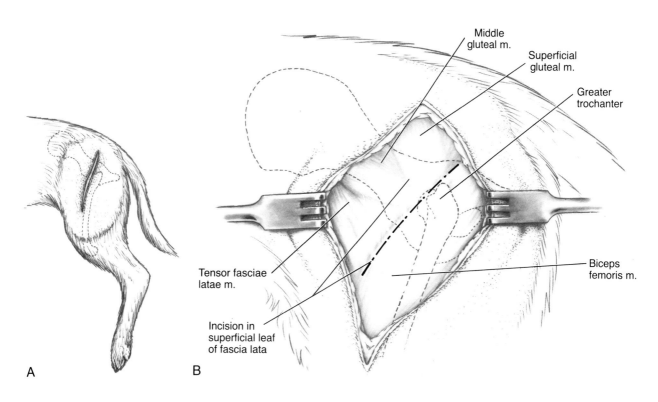

B
Middle gluteal m.
Superficial gluteal m.
Greater trochanter
Tensor fasciae latae m.
Incision in superficial leaf of fascia lata
Biceps femoris m.

A

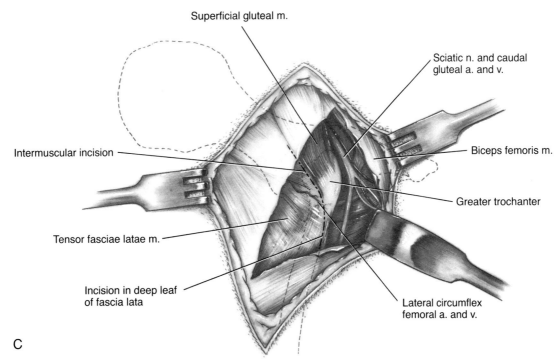

C
Superficial gluteal m.
Sciatic n. and caudal gluteal a. and v.
Intermuscular incision
Biceps femoris m.
Greater trochanter
Tensor fasciae latae m.
Lateral circumflex femoral a. and v.
Incision in deep leaf of fascia lata

Approach to the Craniodorsal Aspect of the Hip Joint Through a Craniolateral Incision *continued*

DESCRIPTION OF THE PROCEDURE *continued*

D. The fascia lata and the attached tensor fasciae latae muscle are retracted cranially and the biceps caudally. Blunt dissection and separation along the neck of the femur with the finger tip allows visualization of a triangle bounded dorsally by the middle and deep gluteal muscles, laterally by the vastus lateralis muscle, and medially by the rectus femoris muscle.

E. The joint capsule is covered by areolar tissue, which must be cleared away by blunt dissection. An incision is then made in the joint capsule and continued laterally along the femoral neck through the origin of the vastus lateralis muscle on the neck and lesser trochanter. Exposure can be improved by tenotomy of a portion of the deep gluteal tendon close to the trochanter, leaving enough tendon on the bone to allow suturing. The muscle is split proximally, parallel to its fibers, and the pedicle is allowed to retract.

Plate 59

Approach to the Craniodorsal Aspect of the Hip Joint Through a Craniolateral Incision *continued*

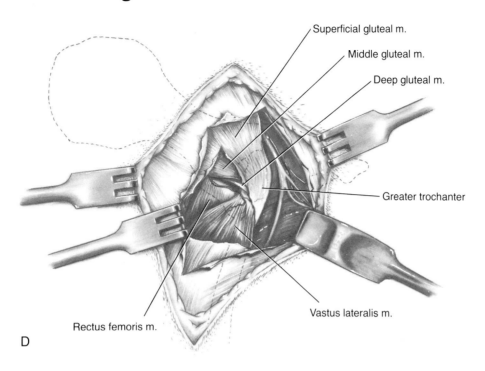

Superficial gluteal m.

Middle gluteal m.

Deep gluteal m.

Greater trochanter

Vastus lateralis m.

Rectus femoris m.

D

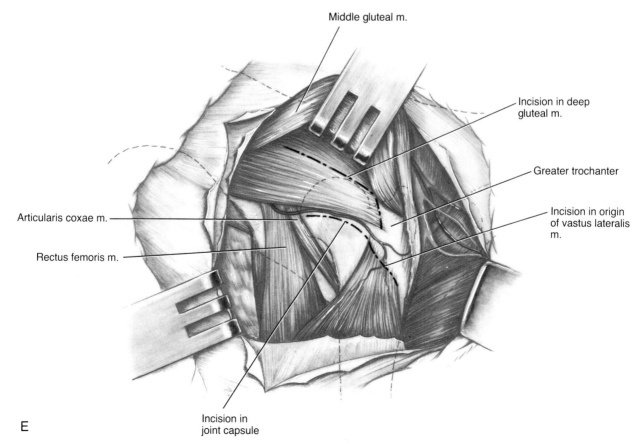

Middle gluteal m.

Incision in deep gluteal m.

Greater trochanter

Incision in origin of vastus lateralis m.

Articularis coxae m.

Rectus femoris m.

Incision in joint capsule

E

Approach to the Craniodorsal Aspect of the Hip Joint Through a Craniolateral Incision *continued*

DESCRIPTION OF THE PROCEDURE *continued*

F. The origin of the vastus lateralis muscle is elevated from the femoral neck and reflected distally. The muscle comes free most easily if the elevation proceeds from distal to proximal. This elevation can be subperiosteal in the immature animal or extraperiosteal in the mature patient. Hohmann retractors are placed intracapsularly ventrally and caudally to the femoral neck, to allow visualization of the femoral head. Caution is needed to be certain that the caudal retractor is intracapsular, or at least between the deep gluteal muscle and the femoral neck, in order to avoid entrapping the sciatic nerve on the caudodorsal surface of the deep gluteal muscle.

CLOSURE

One or two mattress sutures are placed in the deep gluteal tendon incision, and the origin of the vastus lateralis muscle is sutured to the cranial edge of the deep gluteal muscle. Continuous sutures are placed in the insertion of the tensor fasciae latae muscle distally and continued proximally along the cranial border of the superficial gluteal muscle. The superficial leaf of the fascia lata distally and the gluteal fascia proximally are closed to the cranial border of the biceps femoris with a continuous pattern. The rest of the area is closed routinely in layers.

Plate 59

Approach to the Craniodorsal Aspect of the Hip Joint Through a Craniolateral Incision *continued*

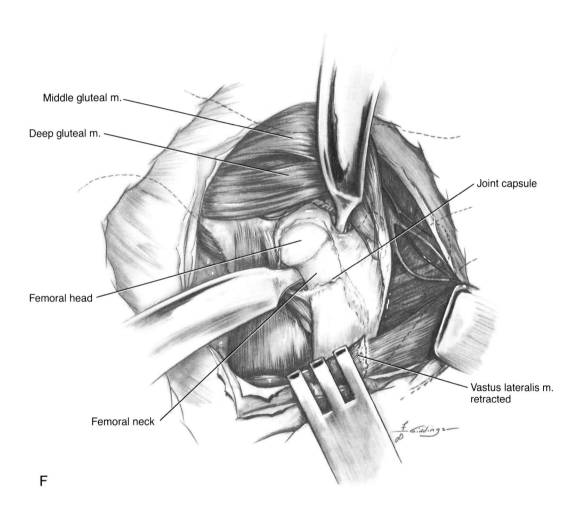

Middle gluteal m.

Deep gluteal m.

Joint capsule

Femoral head

Vastus lateralis m. retracted

Femoral neck

F

Approach to the Dorsal Aspect of the Hip Joint Through an Intergluteal Incision

Based on a Procedure of Wadsworth and Henry[41]

INDICATION

Internal fixation of fractures in the central part of the acetabulum.

ALTERNATIVE/COMBINATION APPROACHES

Plates 59, 61, 62, and 63

DESCRIPTION OF THE PROCEDURE

A. Commencing distal to the greater trochanter of the femur, the skin incision crosses the trochanter and curves in a craniomedial direction proximally, ending about halfway between the trochanter and the dorsal midline.

B. Skin and subcutaneous fat are undermined and retracted to allow visualization of the gluteal fascia, which is incised along the cranial border of the biceps femoris and superficial gluteal muscles. These two incisions meet in the region of the greater trochanter.

Plate 60

Approach to the Dorsal Aspect of the Hip Joint Through an Intergluteal Incision

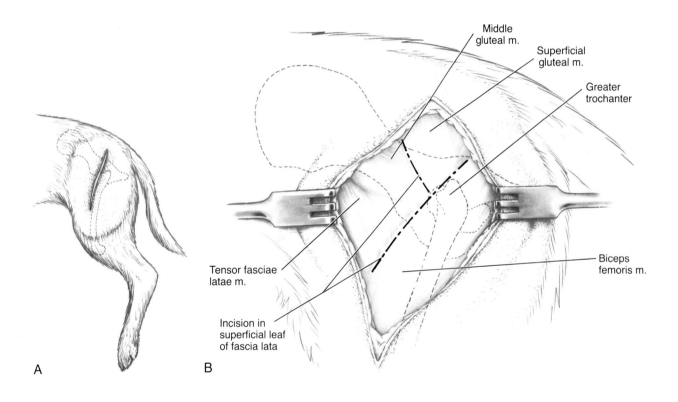

Middle gluteal m.

Superficial gluteal m.

Greater trochanter

Biceps femoris m.

Tensor fasciae latae m.

Incision in superficial leaf of fascia lata

A

B

Approach to the Dorsal Aspect of the Hip Joint Through an Intergluteal Incision *continued*

DESCRIPTION OF THE PROCEDURE *continued*

C. The belly of the superficial gluteal muscle is elevated preparatory to tenotomizing it near its insertion on the third trochanter of the femur. The sciatic nerve will be visualized as this muscle is elevated. Cranial retraction of the middle gluteal muscle results in a separation developing between it and the piriformis muscle (as illustrated), or they may remain attached and retract as a single muscle.

D. Elevation and retraction of the superficial gluteal muscle will allow retraction of the sciatic nerve with a Penrose rubber drain. The origin of the deep gluteal muscle on the shaft of the ilium is incised, starting at its caudal border near the ischiatic spine. This incision continues cranially as needed to allow elevation and retraction of the muscle belly in a craniolateral direction to expose the dorsal rim of the acetabulum. Pointed Hohmann retractors are placed cranial and caudal to the femoral head, the latter serving to retract the internal obturator and gemelli muscles. The joint capsule can be incised now to aid in orientation.

CLOSURE

Interrupted absorbable sutures, size 2/0 or 3/0, are placed in the joint capsule. The deep gluteal muscle is reattached to its origin if any tissue is available for suturing; otherwise, the muscle is simply placed back in position and allowed to heal by fibrosis. Mattress sutures of nonabsorbable material are used in the superficial gluteal tendon; fascia, subcutaneous tissues, and skin are closed routinely in layers.

COMMENTS

Although relatively speedy to perform, this approach gives limited exposure. The fracture must be in the center of the joint and noncomminuted.

Plate 60

Approach to the Dorsal Aspect of the Hip Joint Through an Intergluteal Incision *continued*

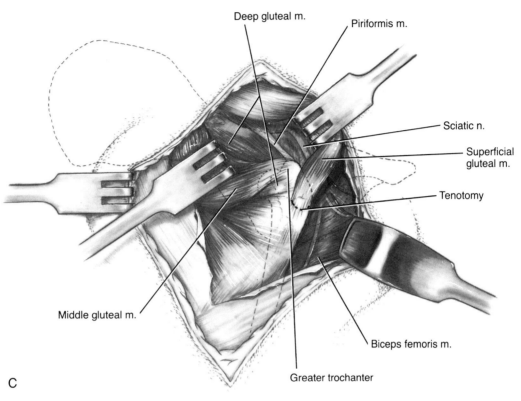

Deep gluteal m.

Piriformis m.

Sciatic n.

Superficial gluteal m.

Tenotomy

Middle gluteal m.

Biceps femoris m.

Greater trochanter

C

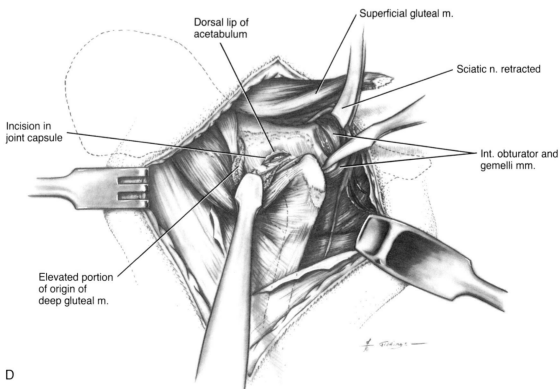

Dorsal lip of acetabulum

Superficial gluteal m.

Sciatic n. retracted

Incision in joint capsule

Int. obturator and gemelli mm.

Elevated portion of origin of deep gluteal m.

D

Approach to the Craniodorsal and Caudodorsal Aspects of the Hip Joint by Osteotomy of the Greater Trochanter

Based on a Procedure of Gorman[13]

INDICATIONS

1. Open reduction of coxofemoral luxations.
2. Open reduction of fractures in the cranial half of the acetabulum or the caudal body of the ilium.
3. Open reduction of fractures of the femoral head and neck (see "Comments" below).
4. Installation of total hip prostheses.

DESCRIPTION OF THE PROCEDURE

A. The skin incision is centered on the cranial aspect of the greater trochanter of the femur, curving craniomedially to near the midline, and following the cranial border of the femur distally to near midshaft. The alternative curved flap incision is preferred by some.

B. Subcutaneous tissues are reflected with the skin. An incision is made in the superficial leaf of the fascia lata along the cranial border of the biceps femoris muscle for the entire length of the exposure.

C. The biceps femoris muscle is retracted caudally and the sciatic nerve identified. An incision is made in the deep leaf of the fascia lata to free the insertion of the tensor fasciae latae muscle. This incision is continued proximally along the cranial border of the superficial gluteal muscle. The tendon of insertion of this muscle is cut close to the third trochanter, leaving enough tissue on the bone to allow suturing.

Plate 61

Approach to the Craniodorsal and Caudodorsal Aspects of the Hip Joint by Osteotomy of the Greater Trochanter

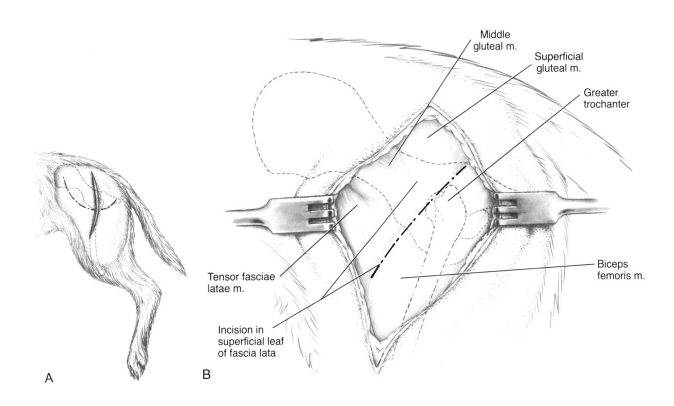

Middle gluteal m.

Superficial gluteal m.

Greater trochanter

Biceps femoris m.

Tensor fasciae latae m.

Incision in superficial leaf of fascia lata

A

B

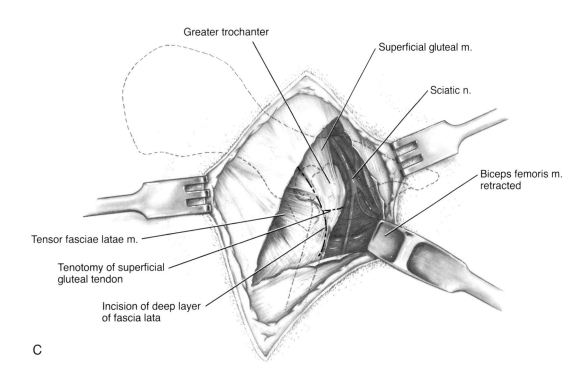

Greater trochanter

Superficial gluteal m.

Sciatic n.

Biceps femoris m. retracted

Tensor fasciae latae m.

Tenotomy of superficial gluteal tendon

Incision of deep layer of fascia lata

C

Approach to the Craniodorsal and Caudodorsal Aspects of the Hip Joint by Osteotomy of the Greater Trochanter *continued*

DESCRIPTION OF THE PROCEDURE *continued*

D, E. The superficial gluteal muscle is retracted craniodorsally. The greater trochanter is osteotomized by placing the osteotome on the lateral surface of the greater trochanter, just proximal to the superficial gluteal muscle insertion on the third trochanter. The osteotome is positioned to form a 45° angle with the long axis of the femur (see E) so as to cut the trochanter flush with the femoral neck beneath the insertions of the middle and deep gluteal muscles. Alternatively, a Gigli wire saw can be used for the osteotomy.

Plate 61

Approach to the Craniodorsal and Caudodorsal Aspects of the Hip Joint by Osteotomy of the Greater Trochanter

continued

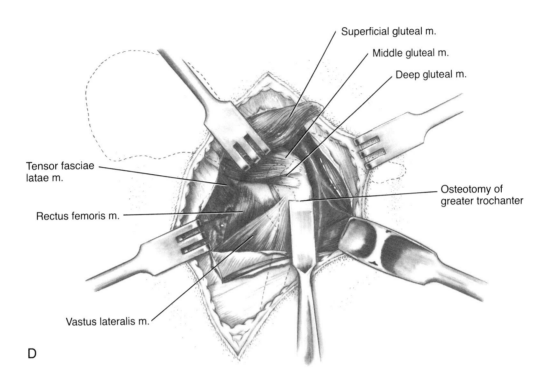

Superficial gluteal m.

Middle gluteal m.

Deep gluteal m.

Tensor fasciae latae m.

Rectus femoris m.

Osteotomy of greater trochanter

Vastus lateralis m.

D

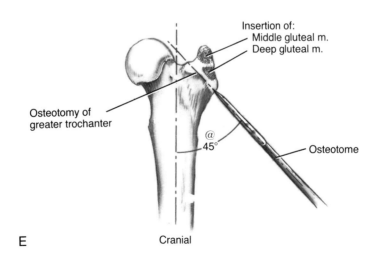

Insertion of:
Middle gluteal m.
Deep gluteal m.

Osteotomy of greater trochanter

@ 45°

Osteotome

E

Cranial

Approach to the Craniodorsal and Caudodorsal Aspects of the Hip Joint by Osteotomy of the Greater Trochanter *continued*

DESCRIPTION OF THE PROCEDURE *continued*

F. The middle and deep gluteal muscles are reflected dorsomedially as a unit with the greater trochanter. The deep gluteal muscle must be sharply dissected from the joint capsule and can then be subperiosteally elevated from the ilium as desired for exposure. The sciatic nerve must be protected during this dissection.

CLOSURE

The greater trochanter is attached to its bed by two Kirschner wires or with the tension band wire technique (Figure 23A). Interrupted sutures are placed in the insertion of the superficial gluteal muscle and continuous sutures in the insertion of the tensor fascia lata muscle. The superficial leaf of the fascia lata distally and the gluteal fascia proximally are closed to the cranial border of the biceps femoris with a continuous pattern. Subcutaneous tissues and skin are closed in separate layers.

COMMENTS

The choice between this approach and the Approach to the Craniodorsal and Caudodorsal Aspects of the Hip Joint by Tenotomy of the Gluteal Muscles (Plate 62) is primarily one of personal preference of the surgeon. There is no difference in the exposure obtained. Although popular for repair of fractures of the femoral neck, adequate exposure can usually be obtained by the Approach to the Craniodorsal Aspect of the Hip Joint Through a Craniolateral Incision (Plate 59), a somewhat quicker procedure.

Plate 61

Approach to the Craniodorsal and Caudodorsal Aspects of the Hip Joint by Osteotomy of the Greater Trochanter

continued

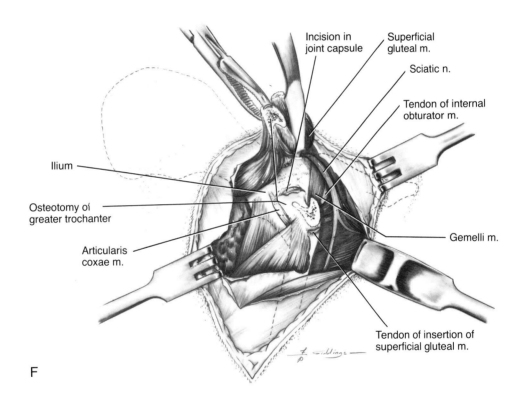

Incision in joint capsule

Superficial gluteal m.

Sciatic n.

Tendon of internal obturator m.

Ilium

Osteotomy of greater trochanter

Articularis coxae m.

Gemelli m.

Tendon of insertion of superficial gluteal m.

F

Approach to the Craniodorsal and Caudodorsal Aspects of the Hip Joint by Tenotomy of the Gluteal Muscles

Based on a Procedure of Brown[5]

INDICATIONS

1. Open reduction of coxofemoral luxations.
2. Open reduction of fractures of the cranial half of the acetabulum or the caudal body of the ilium.
3. Open reduction of fractures of the femoral head and neck (see "Comments" below).
4. Installation of total hip prostheses.

ALTERNATIVE/COMBINATION APPROACHES

Plates 59, 60, 61, 63, and 64

DESCRIPTION OF THE PROCEDURE

This approach is started as depicted in Plate 61, Parts A–C.

A. The superficial gluteal muscle is retracted proximally to expose the middle gluteal muscle, and the belly of this muscle is undermined near its insertion on the trochanter. The tendinous insertion is transected as close as possible to the bone. Protect the sciatic nerve during these procedures.

The freed middle gluteal and attached piriformis muscles are retracted dorsally to allow the deep gluteal muscle to be undermined similarly to the middle gluteal muscle. The insertion of the deep gluteal extends more cranially and distally on the trochanter than does the middle gluteal. A tenotomy is performed close to the bone.

B. Sharp dissection is required to free the deep gluteal muscle from the joint capsule, following which it can be subperiosteally elevated from the ilium as desired for exposure.

CLOSURE

Interrupted sutures are placed in the joint capsule. The tendons of the deep and middle gluteal muscles are reattached to the trochanter by passing suture through holes drilled in the trochanter, as illustrated in Figure 22. Locking-loop or mattress sutures are placed in the tendon of the superficial gluteal muscle, and a continuous layer in the insertion of the tensor fasciae latae muscle. The superficial leaf of the tensor fascia lata distally and the gluteal fascia proximally are closed to the cranial border of the biceps femoris with a continuous pattern.

COMMENTS

Because of the tenotomies, function is not regained as quickly with this approach as with the osteotomy of the greater trochanter (Plate 61). This approach may be preferable to osteotomy in the skeletally immature animal, because there is no disruption of the physis of the greater trochanter.

Plate 62

Approach to the Craniodorsal and Caudodorsal Aspects of the Hip Joint by Tenotomy of the Gluteal Muscles

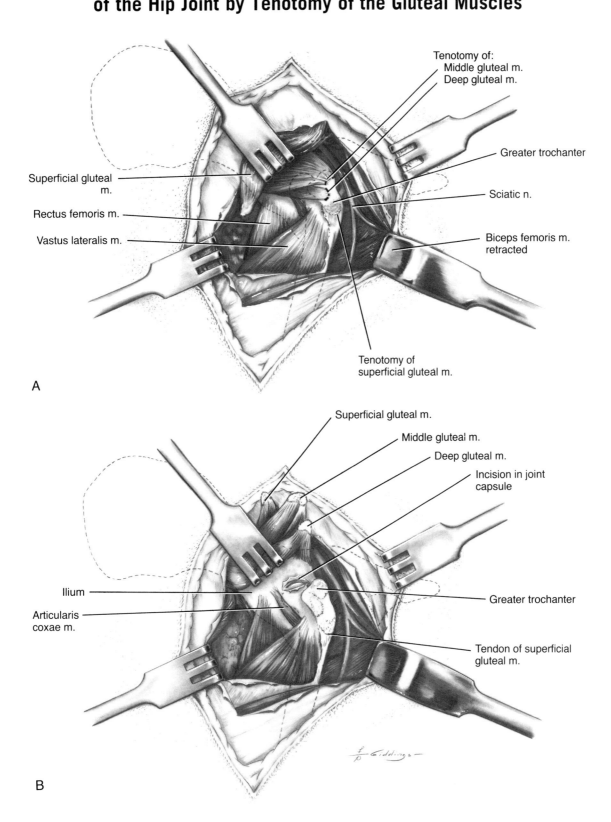

A

B

Approach to the Caudal Aspect of the Hip Joint and Body of the Ischium

Based on Procedures of Hohn[15] and Slocum and Hohn[36]

INDICATIONS

1. Femoral head resection and other arthroplastic procedures.
2. Open reduction of fractures of the caudal region of the acetabulum and of the cranial body of the ischium.
3. Open reduction of craniodorsal coxofemoral luxations.

ALTERNATIVE/COMBINATION APPROACHES

Plates 59, 60, 61, 62, and 64

DESCRIPTION OF THE PROCEDURE

A. The curved incision is centered on the caudal surface of the greater trochanter. It starts near the dorsal midline, continues caudal to the trochanter, and extends through the proximal one fourth to one third of the femur.

B. The subcutaneous fat is undermined and retracted with the skin. The fascia of the biceps muscle is incised at the cranial border of the muscle from the sacrotuberous ligament proximally, and distally to the end of the skin incision.

C. The tendinous insertion of the superficial gluteal muscle is cut near its attachment on the third trochanter, and the incision is continued into the deep leaf of the fascia lata. This muscle is now retracted craniodorsally and the biceps caudally to expose the external rotator muscles of the hip.

Plate 63

Approach to the Caudal Aspect of the Hip Joint and Body of the Ischium

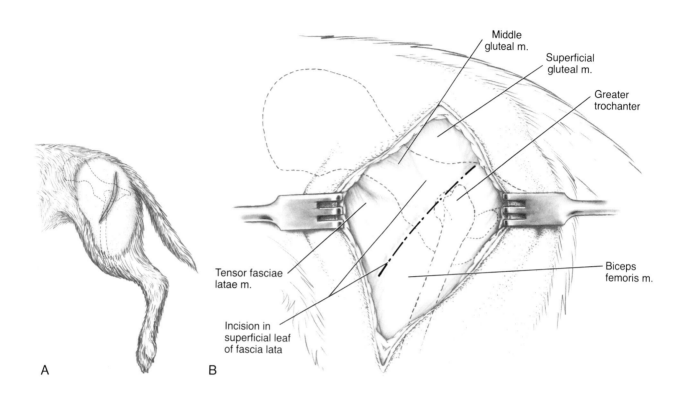

Middle gluteal m.

Superficial gluteal m.

Greater trochanter

Tensor fasciae latae m.

Biceps femoris m.

Incision in superficial leaf of fascia lata

A

B

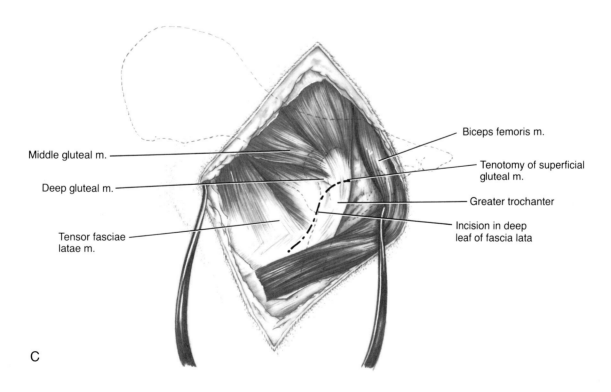

Middle gluteal m.

Deep gluteal m.

Tensor fasciae latae m.

Biceps femoris m.

Tenotomy of superficial gluteal m.

Greater trochanter

Incision in deep leaf of fascia lata

C

Approach to the Caudal Aspect of the Hip Joint and Body of the Ischium *continued*

DESCRIPTION OF THE PROCEDURE *continued*

D. With the femur internally rotated, the combined tendon of insertion of the internal obturator and gemelli muscles is cut close to its attachment in the trochanteric fossa.

E. A stay suture in the tendon of the internal obturator and gemelli muscles will aid in its retraction. As it is retracted, it also retracts and protects the sciatic nerve as the obturator fossa of the ischium is exposed. Dissection of a portion of the origin of the deep gluteal muscle will enhance the exposure of the caudodorsal labrum of the acetabulum. A Hohmann retractor placed ventral to the femoral head will help retract the external obturator and quadratus muscles. Care must be taken to protect the sciatic nerve and circumflex femoral vessels.

CLOSURE

Nonabsorbable suture is used to place a modified Bunnell-Mayer or locking-loop suture (Figure 21A, C) in the tendon of the internal obturator and gemelli muscles. It is usually impossible to suture to the small portion of the insertion that remains in the trochanteric fossa, so the suture is attached to the insertions of the deep and middle gluteal muscles at the trochanter. Alternatively, twin holes can be drilled through the femoral neck as illustrated in Plate 64, Part D, and the suture is passed through these holes and tied.

COMMENTS

When used in the open reduction of a craniodorsal coxofemoral luxation, this approach provides good exposure of the acetabulum, allowing it to be easily cleaned of debris before reduction is attempted. In these situations, this approach can be combined with the Approach to the Craniodorsal and Caudodorsal Aspects of the Hip Joint by Osteotomy of the Greater Trochanter (Plate 61).

Plate 63

Approach to the Caudal Aspect of the Hip Joint and Body of the Ischium *continued*

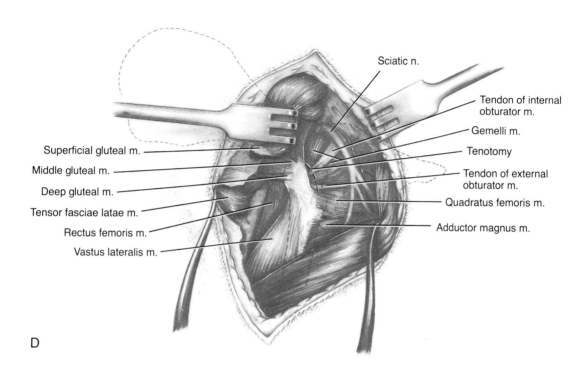

Sciatic n.

Tendon of internal obturator m.

Gemelli m.

Tenotomy

Tendon of external obturator m.

Quadratus femoris m.

Adductor magnus m.

Superficial gluteal m.

Middle gluteal m.

Deep gluteal m.

Tensor fasciae latae m.

Rectus femoris m.

Vastus lateralis m.

D

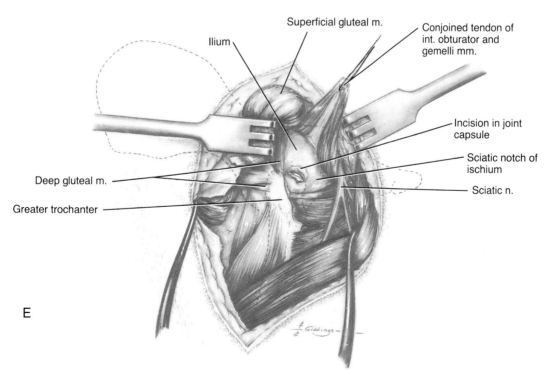

Superficial gluteal m.

Ilium

Conjoined tendon of int. obturator and gemelli mm.

Incision in joint capsule

Sciatic notch of ischium

Sciatic n.

Deep gluteal m.

Greater trochanter

E

Approach to the Os Coxae

INDICATION

Open reduction and internal fixation of multiple fractures of the hemipelvis.

EXPLANATORY NOTE

This procedure combines elements of three approaches: Approach to the Ilium Through a Lateral Incision (Plate 57), Approach to the Craniodorsal and Caudodorsal Aspects of the Hip Joint by Osteotomy of the Greater Trochanter (Plate 61), and Approach to the Caudal Aspect of the Hip Joint and Body of the Ischium (Plate 63). They should be studied before proceeding.

DESCRIPTION OF THE PROCEDURE

A. The skin incision begins near the center of the iliac crest, runs caudally to a point distal to the greater trochanter of the femur, and then curves dorsally to end near the ischiatic tuberosity. Subcutaneous tissues and gluteal fascia are incised along the same line as the skin. Additional gluteal fascial incisions are made as shown in Plate 57, Part B, and Plate 61, Parts B and C. The superficial gluteal muscle is tenotomized near its insertion and the greater trochanter is osteotomized as in Plate 61, Parts D and E.

B. Middle and deep gluteal muscles are elevated from the wing and shaft of the ilium and reflected dorsomedially with the trochanter. This is sufficient exposure for the iliac shaft and cranial acetabular areas.

C, D. For exposure of the caudal acetabular and ischial regions, the combined tendon of the internal obturator and gemelli muscles is cut at its insertion in the trochanteric fossa. Caudomedial retraction of these muscles protects the sciatic nerve and exposes the region of the ischiatic notch. Note that the modified Bunnell-Mayer suture to be used in closure has been inserted in the tendon to aid in retraction of these muscles.

CLOSURE

Illustration D shows how the internal obturator/gemelli tendon is attached to the femoral neck. Two holes drilled through the femoral neck allow the tendon to be securely approximated. The greater trochanter is attached to the femur by means of Kirschner wires and tension band wire (see Figure 23A). The tendon of the superficial gluteal muscle is sutured to its insertion of the third trochanter. Fascial incisions, subcutaneous tissues, and skin are closed in separate layers.

Plate 64
Approach to the Os Coxae

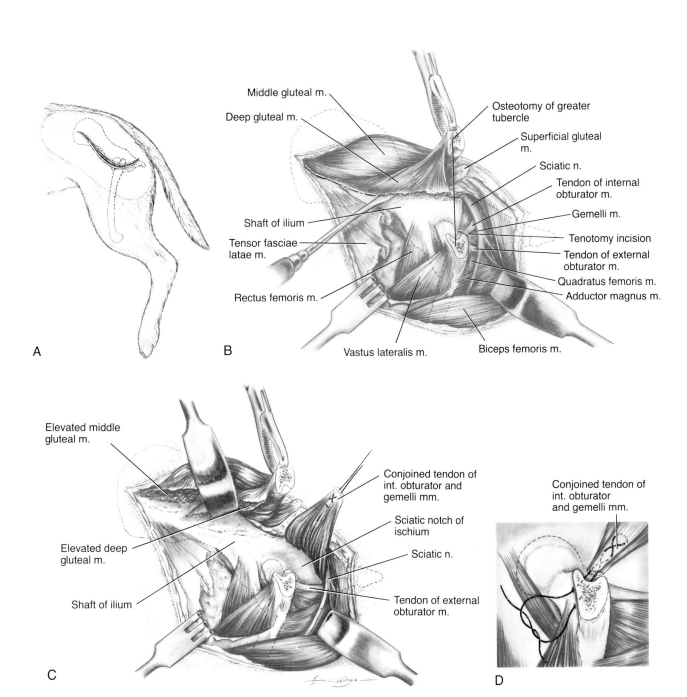

B
- Middle gluteal m.
- Deep gluteal m.
- Osteotomy of greater tubercle
- Superficial gluteal m.
- Sciatic n.
- Tendon of internal obturator m.
- Shaft of ilium
- Gemelli m.
- Tenotomy incision
- Tensor fasciae latae m.
- Tendon of external obturator m.
- Quadratus femoris m.
- Adductor magnus m.
- Rectus femoris m.
- Vastus lateralis m.
- Biceps femoris m.

A

C
- Elevated middle gluteal m.
- Conjoined tendon of int. obturator and gemelli mm.
- Sciatic notch of ischium
- Elevated deep gluteal m.
- Sciatic n.
- Shaft of ilium
- Tendon of external obturator m.

D
- Conjoined tendon of int. obturator and gemelli mm.

Approach to the Ventral Aspect of the Hip Joint or the Ramus of the Pubis

Based on Procedures of Hohn[15] and Slocum and Devine[35]

INDICATIONS

1. Open reduction of ventral luxations of the femoral head.
2. Open reduction of fractures of the ventral aspect of the acetabulum.
3. Ostectomy of the femoral head and neck.
4. Ostectomy of the ramus of the pubis for triple pelvic osteotomy.

DESCRIPTION OF THE PROCEDURE

A. The skin incision is made over the cranial border of the pectineus muscle, starting at the ventral lip of the acetabulum. The incision runs distally along the pectineus for a distance of one third the length of the femur.

B. The fascia is opened in line with the skin incision and the skin flaps undermined and retracted. The belly of the pectineus muscle is mobilized by blunt dissection, with care being taken to protect the femoral artery, vein, and saphenous nerve that run along the cranial border of the muscle. The pectineus is transected near its origin on the prepubic tendon.

C. The pectineus muscle is reflected distally to reveal the iliopsoas muscle and the medial circumflex femoral artery and vein that run caudally and medially to the acetabular portion of the pelvis. It may be necessary to free these vessels from the surrounding fascia and to retract them proximally. Small branches from these vessels may be disrupted during retraction.

Plate 65

Approach to the Ventral Aspect of the Hip Joint or the Ramus of the Pubis

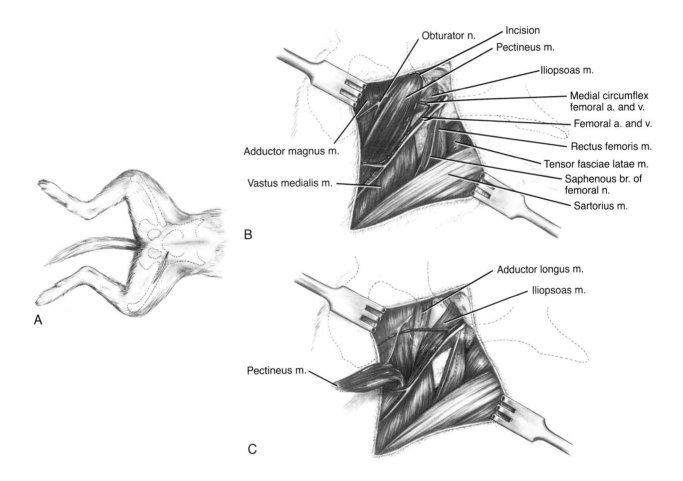

B

Obturator n.
Incision
Pectineus m.
Iliopsoas m.
Medial circumflex femoral a. and v.
Femoral a. and v.
Rectus femoris m.
Tensor fasciae latae m.
Saphenous br. of femoral n.
Sartorius m.
Adductor magnus m.
Vastus medialis m.

A

C

Adductor longus m.
Iliopsoas m.
Pectineus m.

Approach to the Ventral Aspect of the Hip Joint or the Ramus of the Pubis *continued*

DESCRIPTION OF THE PROCEDURE *continued*

D. *If only the pubic ramus is to be exposed, go directly to Part E.* An interval between the iliopsoas and the adductor longus muscle is developed by blunt dissection. Retraction of the iliopsoas cranially and the adductor caudally exposes the rim of the acetabulum. The joint capsule is shown incised so as to reveal the femoral head. Best exposure of the neck of the femur can be developed by placing Hohmann retractors cranial and caudal to the femoral neck.

E. Exposure of the ramus of the pubis is accomplished by retraction of the iliopsoas muscle with a Hohmann retractor placed craniomedially to the iliopectineal eminence. Some of the origin of the adductor longus muscle is elevated from the ramus and another retractor is placed in the obturator foramen. Care must be taken to prevent trapping the obturator nerve between the retractor and the bone.

CLOSURE

Mattress sutures of nonabsorbable material are used to attach the pectineus tendon to the prepubic tendon. A layered closure follows. Alternatively, the muscle can be transected as far distally as possible and the muscle discarded. This is usually done in the triple pelvic osteotomy procedure.

COMMENTS

Exposure of the joint by this approach is quite sparse, and its use is therefore quite limited, although some consider it the approach of choice for femoral head excision because the integrity of the structures dorsal to the joint is maintained.

Plate 65

Approach to the Ventral Aspect of the Hip Joint or the Ramus of the Pubis *continued*

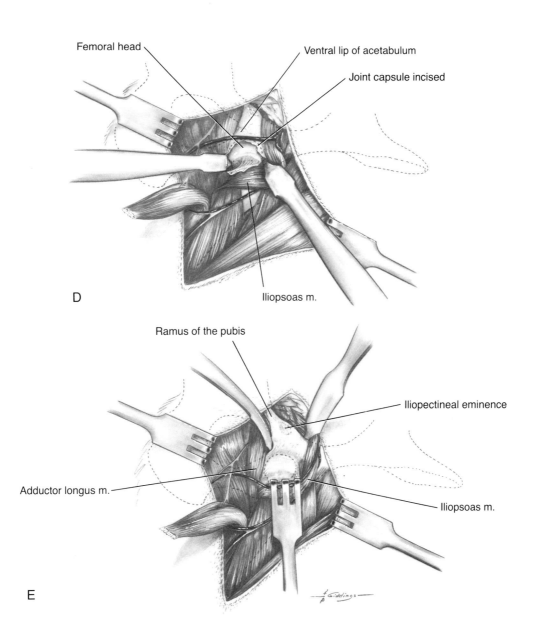

D

Femoral head

Ventral lip of acetabulum

Joint capsule incised

Iliopsoas m.

E

Ramus of the pubis

Iliopectineal eminence

Adductor longus m.

Iliopsoas m.

Approach to the Pubis and Pelvic Symphysis

INDICATIONS

1. Open reduction of fractures of the pubis.
2. Pubic symphysiotomy.

DESCRIPTION OF THE PROCEDURE

A. The skin incision on a male dog is made alongside the penis and extends from the scrotum to a point 1 inch (2.5 cm) cranial to the pubis. In the female dog and cat, the incision is made from the vulva cranially on the midline. The latter technique can also be applied to the male cat.

B. The penis is retracted past the midline, following the incision of the fascia alongside the penis and blunt dissection under the organ. A large branch of the external pudendal artery must be ligated to make the fascial incision.

C. Deep fascia and fat are incised and retracted.

Plate 66

Approach to the Pubis and Pelvic Symphysis

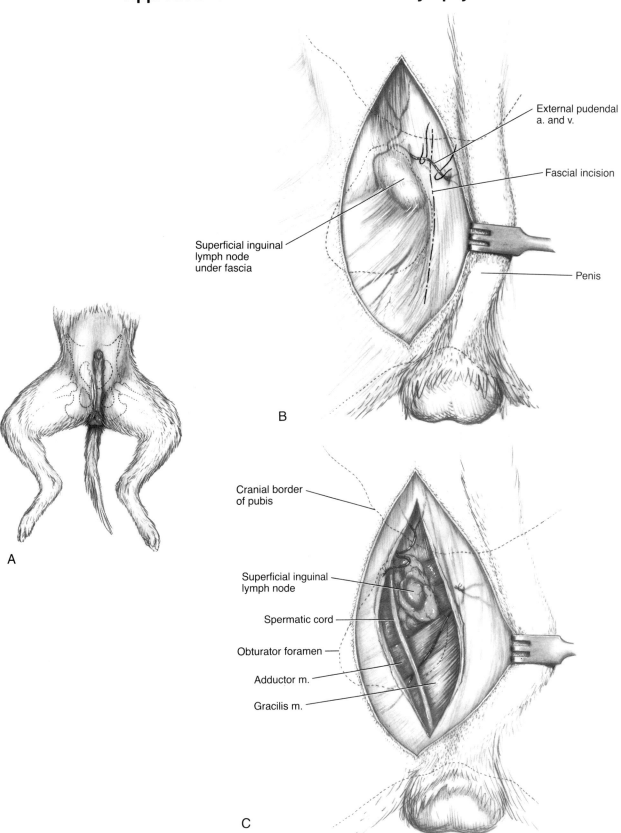

External pudendal
a. and v.

Fascial incision

Superficial inguinal
lymph node
under fascia

Penis

B

A

Cranial border
of pubis

Superficial inguinal
lymph node

Spermatic cord

Obturator foramen

Adductor m.

Gracilis m.

C

Approach to the Pubis and Pelvic Symphysis *continued*

DESCRIPTION OF THE PROCEDURE *continued*

D. A midline incision commencing just cranial to the pubis is made through the linea alba and continued caudally through the subpelvic tendon to the surface of the pubic symphysis.

E. The gracilis and adductor muscles are elevated from the pubic symphysis. Avoid opening the peritoneum if possible.

CLOSURE

The gracilis and adductor muscles are joined at the symphysis by sutures. Any disruption of the insertion of the prepubic tendons must be securely sutured. Attachment to the fascia of the adductor and gracilis muscles is satisfactory. Care must be taken to ensure closure of the peritoneum cranially to the pubis if the peritoneum has been disrupted.

COMMENTS

Excessive abduction of the hindlegs should be prevented for several days by loosely hobbling the legs together.

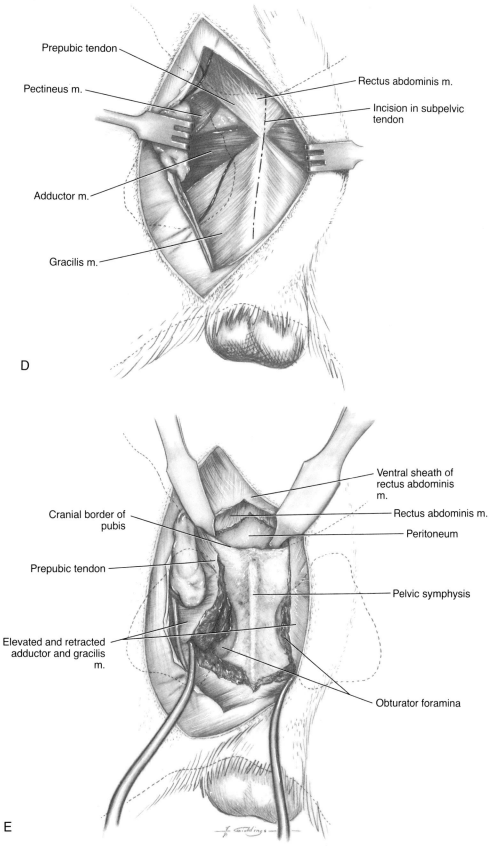

Plate 66

Approach to the Pubis and Pelvic Symphysis *continued*

Prepubic tendon

Pectineus m.

Adductor m.

Gracilis m.

Rectus abdominis m.

Incision in subpelvic tendon

D

Cranial border of pubis

Prepubic tendon

Elevated and retracted adductor and gracilis m.

Ventral sheath of rectus abdominis m.

Rectus abdominis m.

Peritoneum

Pelvic symphysis

Obturator foramina

E

Approach to the Ischium

INDICATIONS

1. Open reduction of fractures of the ischium.
2. Osteotomy of the ramus for triple pelvic osteotomy.

ALTERNATIVE/COMBINATION APPROACHES

Plates 60 through 63

DESCRIPTION OF THE PROCEDURE

A. For exposure of *fractures*, the skin incision is made over the sacrotuberous ligament (absent in cats), which is located by palpation. The incision extends from the level of the greater trochanter to the ischiatic tuberosity. For *osteotomy of the ramus*, the incision is parallel to the midline, starting caudally at the medial angle of the ischiatic tuberosity and extending cranially only half the distance to the level of the greater trochanter (for osteotomy only, go directly to Part D).

B. For exposure of the cranial aspect of the spine of the ischium and visualization of the sciatic nerve, an intermuscular incision is made between the superficial gluteal muscle and the biceps femoris muscle.

C. Caudal retraction of the biceps femoris muscle and cranial retraction of the superficial gluteal muscle provides good exposure of the spine of the ischium and the sciatic nerve.

D. To expose the entire ramus of the ischium, the caudal edge of the origin of the internal obturator muscle is elevated cranially from the table surface until the obturator foramen is visible.

CLOSURE

The elevated internal obturator muscle is sutured to fascia and remnants of periosteum along the ramus. The rest of the incisions are closed in layers.

Plate 67
Approach to the Ischium

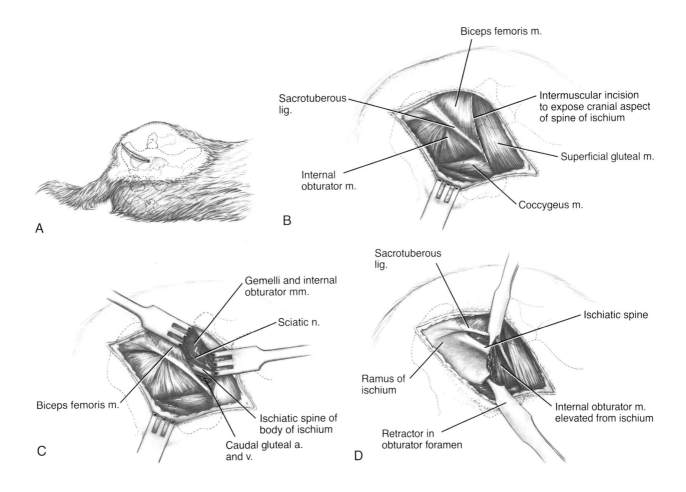

A

B
Biceps femoris m.
Sacrotuberous lig.
Intermuscular incision to expose cranial aspect of spine of ischium
Superficial gluteal m.
Internal obturator m.
Coccygeus m.

C
Gemelli and internal obturator mm.
Sciatic n.
Biceps femoris m.
Ischiatic spine of body of ischium
Caudal gluteal a. and v.

D
Sacrotuberous lig.
Ischiatic spine
Ramus of ischium
Internal obturator m. elevated from ischium
Retractor in obturator foramen

The Hindlimb

- Approach to the Greater Trochanter and Subtrochanteric Region of the Femur

- Approach to the Shaft of the Femur

- Approach to the Distal Femur and Stifle Joint Through a Lateral Incision

- Approach to the Stifle Joint Through a Lateral Incision

- Approach to the Stifle Joint Through a Medial Incision

- Approach to the Stifle Joint with Bilateral Exposure

- Approach to the Distal Femur and Stifle Joint by Osteotomy of the Tibial Tuberosity

- Approach to the Lateral Collateral Ligament and Caudolateral Part of the Stifle Joint

- Approach to the Stifle Joint by Osteotomy of the Origin of the Lateral Collateral Ligament

- Approach to the Medial Collateral Ligament and Caudomedial Part of the Stifle Joint

- Approach to the Stifle Joint by Osteotomy of the Origin of the Medial Collateral Ligament

- Approach to the Shaft of the Tibia

- Approach to the Lateral Malleolus and Talocrural Joint

- Approach to the Medial Malleolus and Talocrural Joint

- Approach to the Tarsocrural Joint by Osteotomy of the Medial Malleolus

- Approach to the Calcaneus

- Approach to the Calcaneus and Plantar Aspects of the Tarsal Bones

- Approach to the Lateral Bones of the Tarsus

- Approach to the Medial Bones of the Tarsus

- Approach to the Proximal Sesamoid Bones

- Approach to the Phalanges and Interphalangeal Joints

- Approaches to the Metatarsal Bones

Approach to the Greater Trochanter and Subtrochanteric Region of the Femur

INDICATION

Open reduction of fractures in the trochanteric and subtrochanteric regions of the femur.

ALTERNATIVE/COMBINATION APPROACHES

Plates 59, 61, 62, 64, and 69

DESCRIPTION OF THE PROCEDURE

A. The skin incision runs from a point dorsal and slightly cranial to the trochanter, extends over the lateral surface of the trochanter, and ends distally at the proximal one third of the shaft of the femur.

B. The subcutaneous fat and fascia are incised and cleared from the area so that the superficial leaf of the fascia lata can be clearly visualized. An incision is made through the fascia lata along the cranial border of the biceps femoris muscle.

C. The biceps is reflected caudally and the skin and fascia lata cranially. The borders of the superficial gluteal muscle are developed by dissection from the surrounding fascia, and the tendon of insertion of this muscle is cut near the femur. Sufficient tendon is left distally to allow suturing at closure.

Plate 68

Approach to the Greater Trochanter and Subtrochanteric Region of the Femur

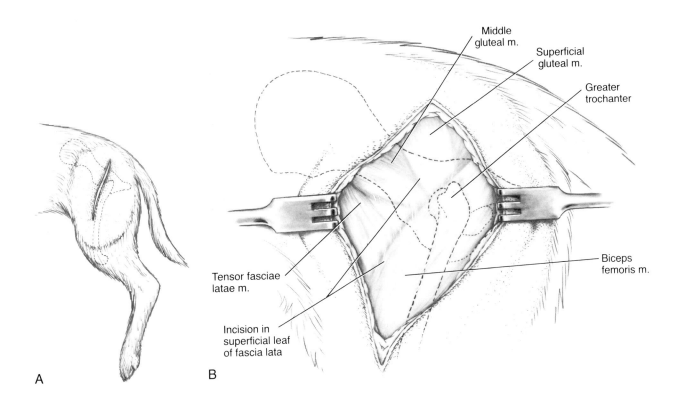

Middle gluteal m.

Superficial gluteal m.

Greater trochanter

Biceps femoris m.

Tensor fasciae latae m.

Incision in superficial leaf of fascia lata

A

B

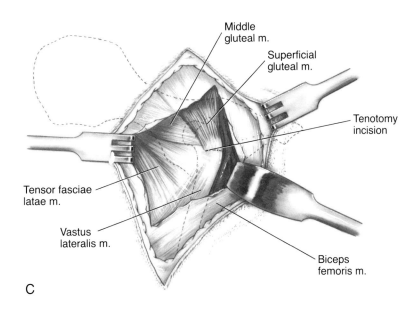

Middle gluteal m.

Superficial gluteal m.

Tenotomy incision

Tensor fasciae latae m.

Vastus lateralis m.

Biceps femoris m.

C

Approach to the Greater Trochanter and Subtrochanteric Region of the Femur *continued*

DESCRIPTION OF THE PROCEDURE *continued*

D. The superficial gluteal muscle is retracted proximally to expose the greater trochanter and the middle gluteal muscle. An incision is now made through the fibers of origin of the vastus lateralis muscle along the ridge of the third trochanter of the femur. This incision is deepened to include the periosteum in young animals.

E. Subperiosteal elevation of this proximal lateral portion of the vastus lateralis muscle exposes the proximal shaft of the femur. The adductor muscle on the caudal side of the bone can also be elevated from the bone to give additional exposure.

CLOSURE

The vastus lateralis muscle is reattached medially to the middle or deep gluteal tendons and laterally to the superficial gluteal tendon. Interrupted mattress sutures are used in the tendon of the superficial gluteal muscle. The fascia lata is then sutured to the biceps femoris, followed by subcutis and skin.

Plate 68

Approach to the Greater Trochanter and Subtrochanteric Region of the Femur *continued*

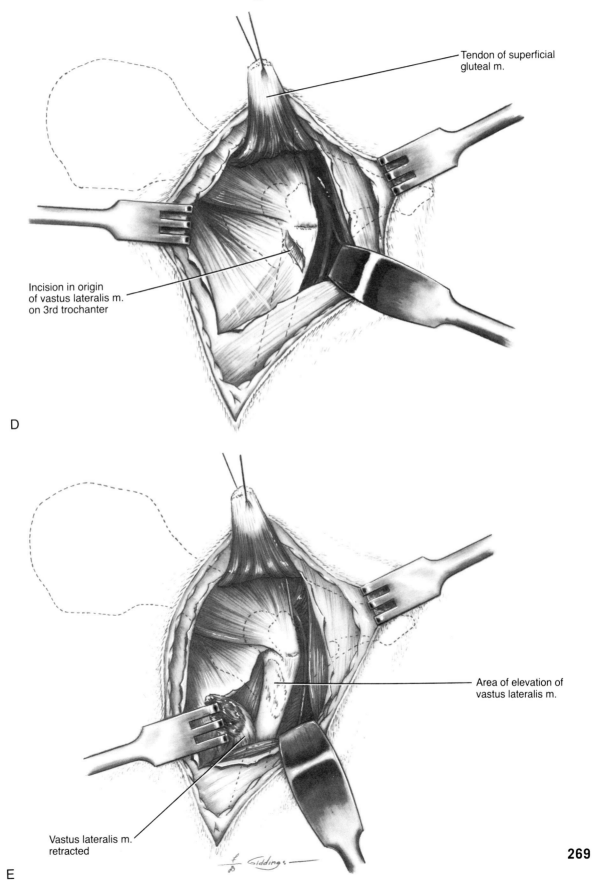

Tendon of superficial gluteal m.

Incision in origin of vastus lateralis m. on 3rd trochanter

D

Area of elevation of vastus lateralis m.

Vastus lateralis m. retracted

E

Approach to the Shaft of the Femur

Based on a Procedure of Brinker[4]

INDICATION

Open reduction of fractures of the femoral shaft proximal to the supracondylar area.

DESCRIPTION OF THE PROCEDURE

A. The skin incision is made along the craniolateral border of the shaft of the bone from the level of the greater trochanter to the level of the patella. The subcutaneous fat and superficial fascia are incised directly under the skin incision.

B. The skin margins are undermined and retracted and the superficial leaf of the fascia lata is incised along the cranial border of the biceps femoris muscle. This incision extends the entire length of the skin incision. If muscle fibers are encountered, the incision should be directed more cranially.

C. Caudal retraction of the biceps femoris reveals the shaft of the femur. It is necessary to incise the fascial aponeurotic septum on the lateral shaft of the bone in order to adequately retract the vastus lateralis.

D. The vastus lateralis and intermedius muscles on the cranial surface of the shaft are retracted by freeing the loose fascia between the muscle and the bone.

CLOSURE

Closure consists of suturing the fascia lata to the cranial border of the biceps muscle in one tier and the subcutaneous fat and fascia in a second tier.

COMMENTS

Limit elevation of the adductor muscle on the caudal one third of the shaft to the extent necessary for visualization of fracture lines, placement of cerclage wires, etc. This muscle is a valuable source of periosteal blood supply to the fracture line caudally.

Plate 69
Approach to the Shaft of the Femur

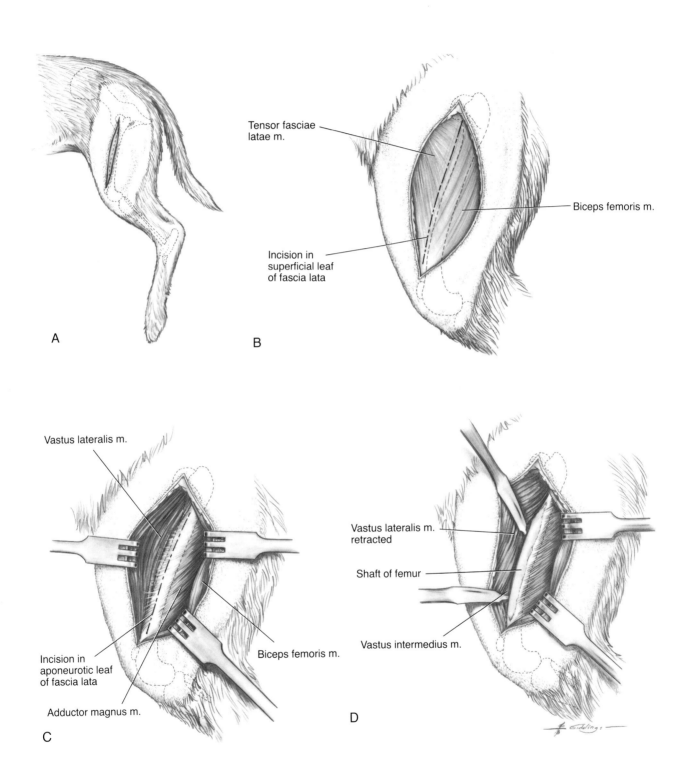

B

Tensor fasciae latae m.

Biceps femoris m.

Incision in superficial leaf of fascia lata

A

C

Vastus lateralis m.

Incision in aponeurotic leaf of fascia lata

Adductor magnus m.

Biceps femoris m.

D

Vastus lateralis m. retracted

Shaft of femur

Vastus intermedius m.

Approach to the Distal Femur and Stifle Joint Through a Lateral Incision

Based on a Procedure of Paatsama[28]

INDICATIONS

1. Open reduction of supracondylar, lateral condylar, intercondylar, and distal physeal fractures of the femur.
2. Exploration of the stifle joint.
3. Medial patellar luxation reconstructions.

ALTERNATIVE/COMBINATION APPROACHES

Plates 69, 71, 72, 73, and 74

DESCRIPTION OF PROCEDURE

A. After palpation of the patella and lateral trochlear ridge, a curved parapatellar skin incision is made extending from the tibial tuberosity to the level of the patella, and then an equal distance proximally. The subcutaneous fascia is incised in the same line as the skin incision. The fascia lata and lateral fascia of the stifle joint are exposed by undermining the subcutaneous fat and fascia, which are then retracted with the skin.

B. Another curved incision, similar to that in the skin, is made through the fascia lata along the cranial border of the biceps. The incision continues distally into the lateral fascia of the stifle joint. As it crosses the trochlear ridge, it curves to parallel the lateral border of the patella and the patellar ligament. Enough fascia is left on the lateral edge of the patella to receive sutures when the joint is closed.

Plate 70

Approach to the Distal Femur and Stifle Joint Through a Lateral Incision

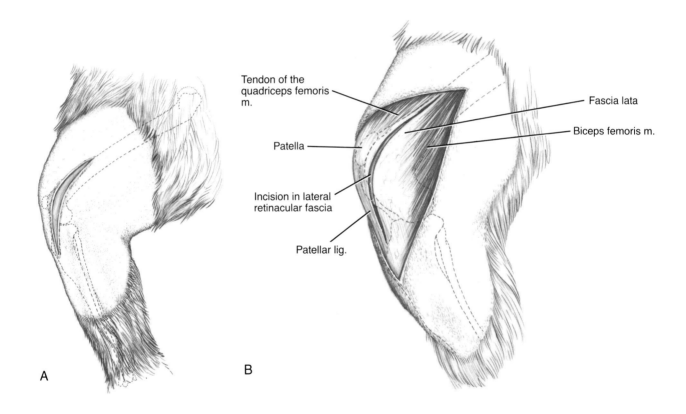

Tendon of the quadriceps femoris m.

Fascia lata

Patella

Biceps femoris m.

Incision in lateral retinacular fascia

Patellar lig.

A

B

Approach to the Distal Femur and Stifle Joint Through a Lateral Incision *continued*

DESCRIPTION OF THE PROCEDURE *continued*

C. The biceps and attached lateral fascia are retracted caudally. In separating the biceps from the vastus lateralis, an intermuscular septum formed from the fascia lata is found attached to the femur. This fascia must be incised to allow mobilization of the quadriceps and biceps. The vessels crossing the area must be ligated in some cases. A parapatellar incision is now made through the joint capsule.

D. With the joint extended, the patella and quadriceps can be luxated medially. Lateral retraction of the joint capsule with the biceps and lateral fascia fully exposes the interior of the joint. Incision and retraction of the infrapatellar fat pad may be necessary for inspection of the menisci and cruciate ligaments.

CLOSURE

The joint capsule and lateral fascia of the stifle joint are closed in one layer with interrupted sutures of nonabsorbable or polydioxanone suture material. Sutures must be placed to prevent any suture material from penetrating the joint capsule in a region where it could abrade articular cartilage. The fascia lata incision proximal to the patella can be closed with a continuous-pattern absorbable suture.

COMMENTS

By combining this approach with the Approach to the Shaft of the Femur (Plate 69), the entire bone can be exposed. It should be noted that the joint capsule usually need not be incised to expose supracondylar fractures, but it is always incised when the fracture is at the physeal line, which is intracapsular. To allow for conversion to bilateral exposure of the joint when needed, this procedure can be done with the animal in dorsal recumbency (see Plate 73).

Plate 70

Approach to the Distal Femur and Stifle Joint
Through a Lateral Incision *continued*

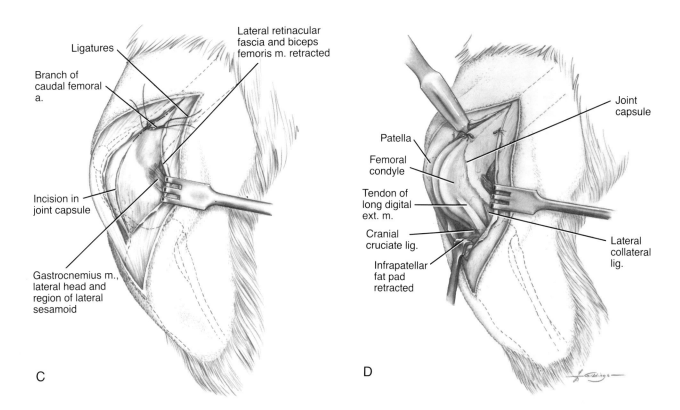

C

- Ligatures
- Branch of caudal femoral a.
- Lateral retinacular fascia and biceps femoris m. retracted
- Incision in joint capsule
- Gastrocnemius m., lateral head and region of lateral sesamoid

D

- Patella
- Femoral condyle
- Tendon of long digital ext. m.
- Cranial cruciate lig.
- Infrapatellar fat pad retracted
- Joint capsule
- Lateral collateral lig.

Approach to the Stifle Joint Through a Lateral Incision

INDICATIONS

1. Cranial cruciate ligament reconstructions.
2. Meniscectomy.
3. Exploration of the stifle joint.

ALTERNATIVE/COMBINATION APPROACHES

Plates 70, 72, 73, 74, and 75

DESCRIPTION OF THE PROCEDURE

A. This approach can be done either in lateral or dorsal recumbency. The skin incision starts over the tibial tuberosity lateral to the patellar ligament, continues proximally to the level of the patella, and then an equal distance proximally following the cranial border of the femur.

B. The arthrotomy incision follows the same line as the skin. The distal portion is made in the lateral fascia first with the scalpel, starting opposite the distal pole of the patella and a few millimeters lateral to the patellar ligament, and continuing distally to the tibia. A stab incision is made into the joint at the proximal end of this incision, which will allow entry into the joint with little danger of damaging articular cartilage of the femoral condyle. One blade of a scissor is inserted into the joint and the scissor is advanced proximally, cutting joint capsule, lateral parapatellar fibrocartilage, and fascia lata. As the proximal part of the incision is started, it is directed slightly laterally so as to cut through the vastus lateralis parallel to the muscle fibers and to leave enough tissue on the lateral side of the patella to permit suturing.

C. The patella can now be luxated medially. If the patella will not stay in position medially, the proximal end of the incision is lengthened. Distal retraction of the fat pad exposes the cruciate ligaments and menisci.

CLOSURE

Distally, the joint capsule and lateral fascia of the stifle joint are closed in one layer with interrupted sutures of nonabsorbable or polydioxanone material. Sutures must be placed so as to prevent any suture material from penetrating the joint in a region where it could abrade articular cartilage. Proximal to the patella the fascia lata can be closed with a continuous-pattern absorbable suture. Subcutis and skin are closed routinely.

COMMENTS

For cosmetic reasons, this skin incision is often made medially, as in Plate 72. The skin can easily be undermined and retracted laterally to make the lateral arthrotomy.

Although this lateral approach is recommended by many for cranial cruciate ligament reconstructions, the author favors a medial approach (see Plate 72), particularly in chronic injuries. These cases often have damage to the caudal horn of the medial meniscus, and meniscectomy is more easily done from the medial side.

Plate 71

Approach to the Stifle Joint Through a Lateral Incision

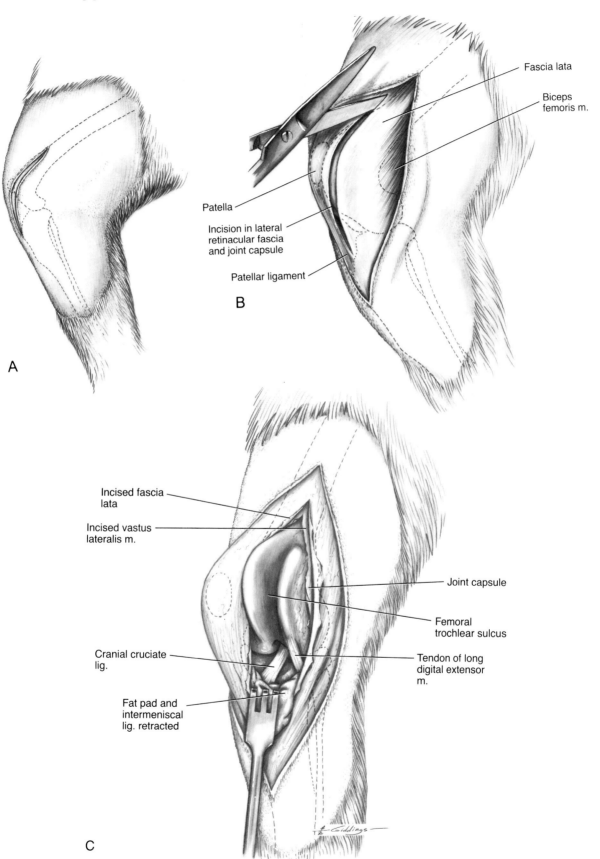

A

B

Fascia lata

Biceps
femoris m.

Patella

Incision in lateral
retinacular fascia
and joint capsule

Patellar ligament

C

Incised fascia
lata

Incised vastus
lateralis m.

Cranial cruciate
lig.

Fat pad and
intermeniscal
lig. retracted

Joint capsule

Femoral
trochlear sulcus

Tendon of long
digital extensor
m.

Approach to the Stifle Joint Through a Medial Incision

INDICATIONS

1. Cranial cruciate ligament reconstructions.
2. Exploration of the stifle joint.
3. Medial meniscectomy.

ALTERNATIVE/COMBINATION APPROACHES

Plates 71, 73, 74, and 77

DESCRIPTION OF THE PROCEDURE

A. The skin incision starts over the tibial tuberosity medial to the patellar ligament, continues proximally to the level of the patella, and then an equal distance proximally following the cranial border of the femur.

B. The arthrotomy incision follows the same line as the skin. The distal portion in the medial fascia is made first with the scalpel, starting opposite the distal pole of the patella and a few millimeters medial to the patellar ligament, and continuing distally to the tibia. A stab incision is made into the joint at the proximal end of this incision, which will allow entry into the joint with little danger of damaging articular cartilage of the femoral condyle. One blade of a scissor is inserted into the joint and the scissor is advanced proximally, cutting joint capsule, medial parapatellar fibrocartilage, medial fascia, and the vastus medialis and cranial part of the sartorius muscles (also see Plate 71, Part B). As the proximal part of the incision is started, it is directed medially so as to cut through the cranial sartorius and vastus medialis muscles parallel to their fibers, and to leave enough tissue on the medial side of the patella to permit suturing.

Plate 72

Approach to the Stifle Joint Through a Medial Incision

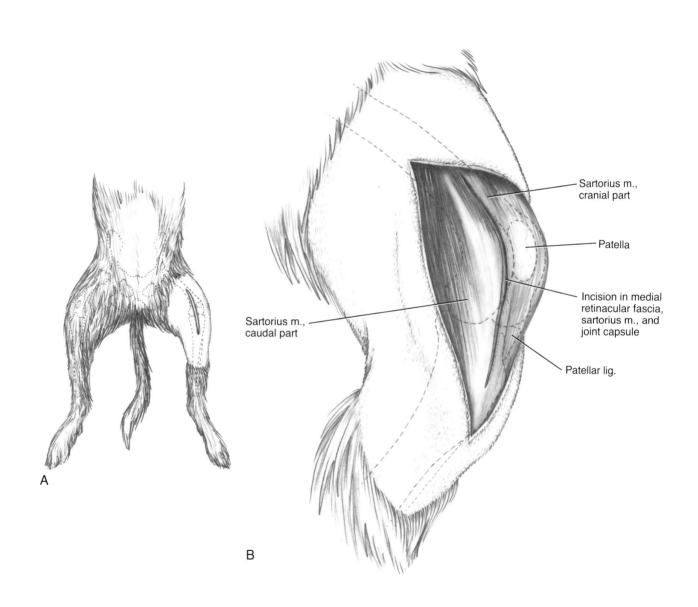

Sartorius m., cranial part

Patella

Incision in medial retinacular fascia, sartorius m., and joint capsule

Patellar lig.

Sartorius m., caudal part

A

B

Approach to the Stifle Joint Through a Medial Incision *continued*

DESCRIPTION OF THE PROCEDURE *continued*

C. The patella can now be luxated laterally. If the patella will not stay in position laterally, the proximal end of the incision is lengthened. Distal retraction of the fat pad exposes the cruciate ligaments and menisci.

CLOSURE

Distally, the joint capsule and medial fascia of the stifle joint are closed in one layer with interrupted sutures of nonabsorbable or polydioxanone material. Sutures must be placed so as to prevent any suture material from penetrating the synovial membrane in a region where it could abrade articular cartilage. Proximal to the patella, the cranial part of the sartorius and the vastus medialis muscles can be closed with a continuous-pattern absorbable suture. Subcutis and skin are closed routinely.

COMMENTS

Medial exposure is preferred over the lateral approach whenever possible. Scar formation is hidden, the interior of the joint is more widely exposed, and medial meniscectomy is more readily performed through a medial incision.

Plate 72

Approach to the Stifle Joint Through a Medial Incision

continued

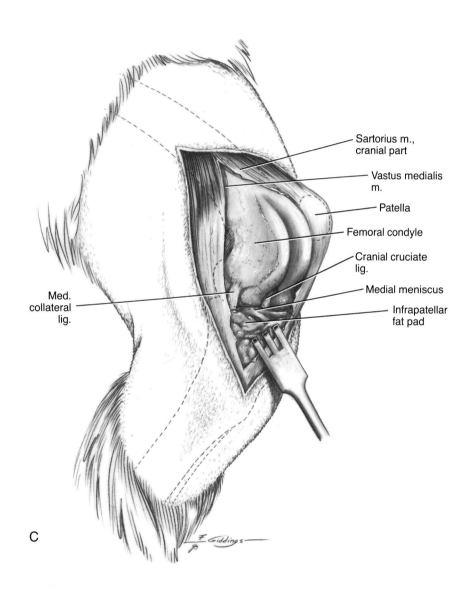

Sartorius m., cranial part

Vastus medialis m.

Patella

Femoral condyle

Cranial cruciate lig.

Medial meniscus

Infrapatellar fat pad

Med. collateral lig.

C

Approach to the Stifle Joint with Bilateral Exposure

INDICATIONS

1. Open reduction of fractures of the distal femur.
2. Double Rush pin fixation of the femur.

DESCRIPTION OF THE PROCEDURE

This procedure is a combination of the Approach to the Distal Femur and Stifle Joint Through a Lateral Incision and the Approach to the Stifle Joint Through a Medial Incision (see Plates 70 and 72).

A. The skin incision is as shown in Plate 70, Part A, although slightly elongated proximally to allow for easier retraction to the medial side. The skin and subcutis are undermined and retracted medially sufficiently to allow access to the medial arthrotomy. If desirable, the skin incision can be placed medially as in Plate 72, Part A, again lengthened proximally to allow easier retraction to the lateral side.

B. Entrance to the lateral side is shown in Parts B, C, and D of Plate 70.

Plate 73
Approach to the Stifle Joint with Bilateral Exposure

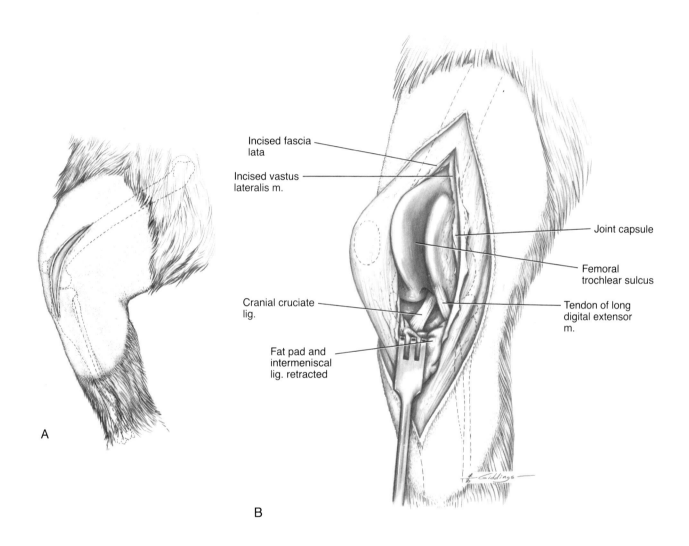

Incised fascia lata

Incised vastus lateralis m.

Joint capsule

Femoral trochlear sulcus

Cranial cruciate lig.

Tendon of long digital extensor m.

Fat pad and intermeniscal lig. retracted

A

B

Approach to the Stifle Joint with Bilateral Exposure *continued*

DESCRIPTION OF THE PROCEDURE *continued*

C. To expose the medial side, see Parts B and C of Plate 72.

D. The entire condylar and supracondylar portion of the femur and the cranial compartment of the stifle joint are now exposed.

CLOSURE

Suturing is done as previously explained for the medial and lateral approaches.

Plate 73

Approach to the Stifle Joint with Bilateral Exposure
continued

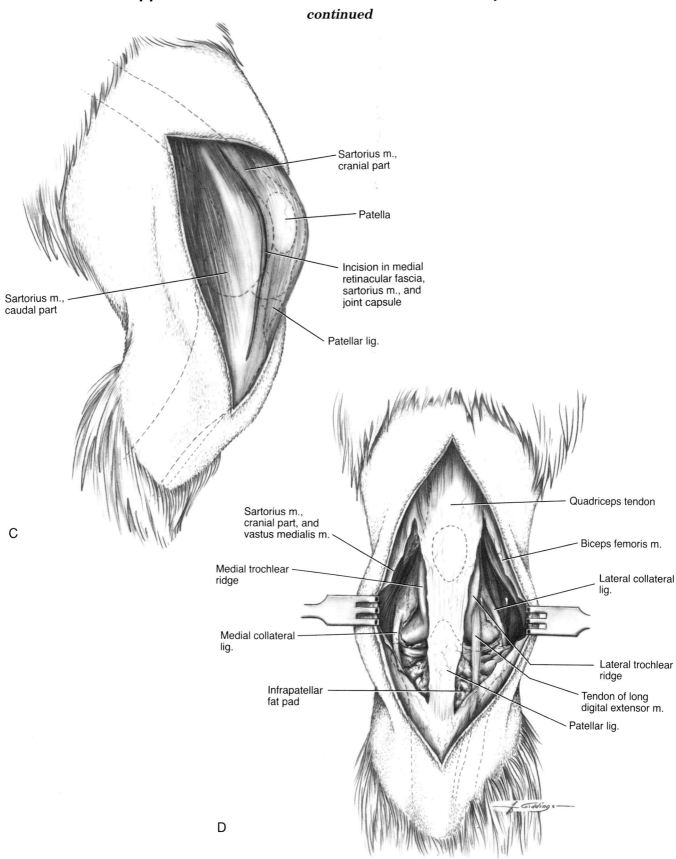

Sartorius m., cranial part

Patella

Incision in medial retinacular fascia, sartorius m., and joint capsule

Patellar lig.

Sartorius m., caudal part

C

Sartorius m., cranial part, and vastus medialis m.

Medial trochlear ridge

Medial collateral lig.

Infrapatellar fat pad

Quadriceps tendon

Biceps femoris m.

Lateral collateral lig.

Lateral trochlear ridge

Tendon of long digital extensor m.

Patellar lig.

D

Approach to the Distal Femur and Stifle Joint by Osteotomy of the Tibial Tuberosity

Based on a Procedure of Nunamaker[25]

INDICATIONS

Open reduction of multiple fractures of the femoral condyles or supracondylar region.

DESCRIPTION OF THE PROCEDURE

This procedure is a modification of the Approach to the Stifle Joint with Bilateral Exposure (Plate 73).

A. An osteotome or Gigli wire saw is used to remove the tibial tuberosity, containing the insertion of the patellar ligament, from the tibia. Care must be exercised to damage neither the articular cartilage of the femoral condyles nor the meniscal cartilages while performing this osteotomy.

B. The detached tibial tuberosity, patellar ligament, and patella are now reflected proximally to expose the femoral condyles, cruciate ligaments, and menisci. If the supracondylar area of the femur must also be exposed, the medial and lateral incisions can be extended proximally as needed.

CLOSURE

The tibial tuberosity is attached to the tibia with Kirschner wires and tension band wire (Figure 23). Subcutaneous tissues and skin are closed in layers. The medial and lateral joint capsules and fascia are closed in one layer, using nonabsorbable or polydioxanone suture material in an interrupted pattern. Fasciae of the quadriceps and biceps muscles are sutured with a continuous pattern and absorbable material.

Plate 74

Approach to the Distal Femur and Stifle Joint by Osteotomy of the Tibial Tuberosity

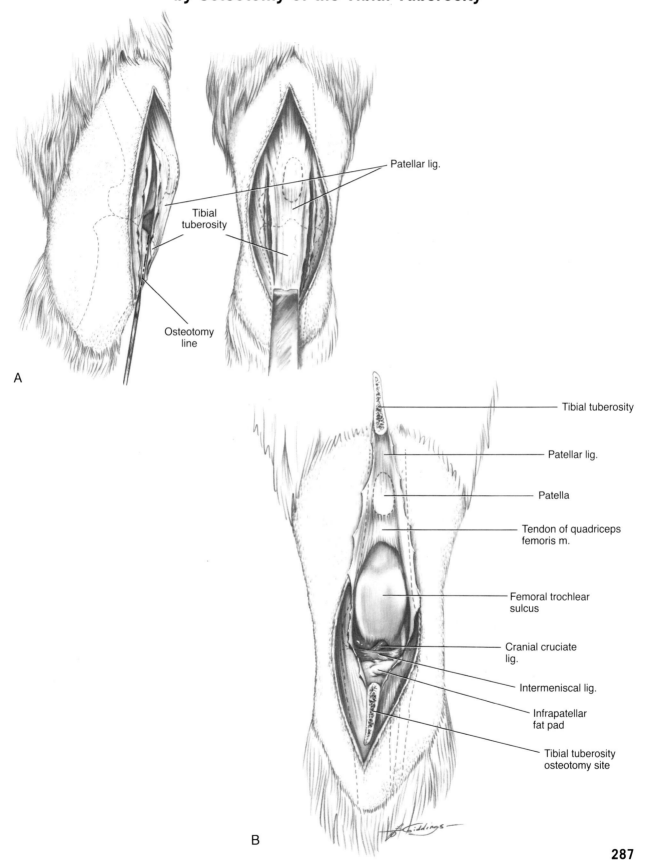

Patellar lig.

Tibial tuberosity

Osteotomy line

A

Tibial tuberosity

Patellar lig.

Patella

Tendon of quadriceps femoris m.

Femoral trochlear sulcus

Cranial cruciate lig.

Intermeniscal lig.

Infrapatellar fat pad

Tibial tuberosity osteotomy site

B

Approach to the Lateral Collateral Ligament and Caudolateral Part of the Stifle Joint

INDICATIONS

1. Removal of the caudal horn of the lateral meniscus.
2. Repair of the lateral collateral ligament or tendon of the popliteus muscle.
3. Open reduction of fractures of the caudal articular surface of the lateral femoral condyle.

ALTERNATIVE/COMBINATION APPROACHES

Plates 70, 71, 73, and 74

DESCRIPTION OF THE PROCEDURE

A. The skin incision is made directly over the distal femur and proximal tibia. The incision commences at the lower third of the femur and continues distally through the proximal fourth of the tibia.

B. Subcutaneous tissues are incised on the same line and retracted with the skin. An incision is made in the aponeurosis of the biceps femoris muscle just cranial to the muscle fibers. It is not necessary to penetrate the joint capsule, although this may be preferable in order to visualize the cranial compartment of the joint (see Plate 70, Part C).

C. As the biceps muscle and attached fascia lata are undermined and retracted caudally, the lateral collateral ligament and tendon of the popliteus muscle are exposed, although still covered by fascia. Note the position of the peroneal nerve and protect it from excessive tension.

D. The caudolateral compartment of the joint is exposed by incising the joint capsule caudally from the collateral ligament. The popliteal tendon and a portion of the joint capsule are elevated to increase exposure. Take care not to damage the meniscus in making this incision.

CLOSURE

Interrupted absorbable sutures are placed in the joint capsule. The aponeurosis of the biceps femoris and the rest of the lateral fascia are closed with either continuous absorbable or interrupted nonabsorbable sutures. Closure of subcutaneous tissues and skin is routine.

Plate 75

Approach to the Lateral Collateral Ligament and Caudolateral Part of the Stifle Joint

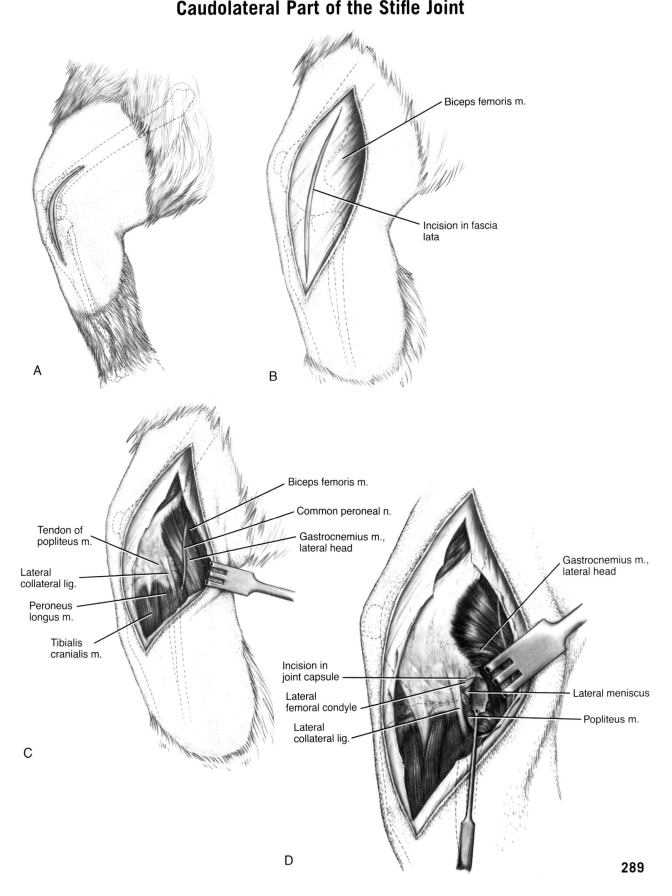

Biceps femoris m.

Incision in fascia lata

A

B

Tendon of popliteus m.

Lateral collateral lig.

Peroneus longus m.

Tibialis cranialis m.

Biceps femoris m.

Common peroneal n.

Gastrocnemius m., lateral head

C

Gastrocnemius m., lateral head

Incision in joint capsule

Lateral femoral condyle

Lateral collateral lig.

Lateral meniscus

Popliteus m.

D

Approach to the Stifle Joint by Osteotomy of the Origin of the Lateral Collateral Ligament

INDICATIONS

1. Reduction of fractures of the caudal part of the lateral femoral condyle.
2. Exploration of the caudolateral part of the stifle joint.
3. Avulsion of the insertion of the caudal cruciate ligament.

ALTERNATIVE/COMBINATION APPROACHES

Plates 70, 71, 74, and 75

DESCRIPTION OF THE PROCEDURE

This procedure is a continuation of the Approach to the Lateral Collateral Ligament and Caudolateral Part of the Stifle Joint (Plate 75).

A. Incision of the joint capsule is continued cranially after elevating the lateral collateral ligament from the joint capsule and lateral retinaculum. This will expose the tendon of the popliteus muscle and its insertion on the femoral condyle. An osteotome is used to outline a block of bone that contains the entire origin of the lateral collateral ligament.

B. The block of bone is freed from the underlying condyle. Be sure to take an adequate amount of bone, because too small a block is difficult to fix securely in place. Note the wedge shape of the bone block; this will have some inherent stability when replaced. Adduction and internal rotation of the tibia will expose the interior of the joint.

CLOSURE

The bone block origin of the ligament is reattached to the femur by means of a lag screw (Figure 24A). This can be simplified by predrilling before cutting the bone block. Interrupted sutures are placed in the joint capsule. The aponeurosis of the biceps femoris and the rest of the lateral fascia are closed with either continuous absorbable or interrupted nonabsorbable sutures. Closure of the subcutaneous tissues and skin is routine.

Plate 76

Approach to the Stifle Joint by Osteotomy of the Origin of the Lateral Collateral Ligament

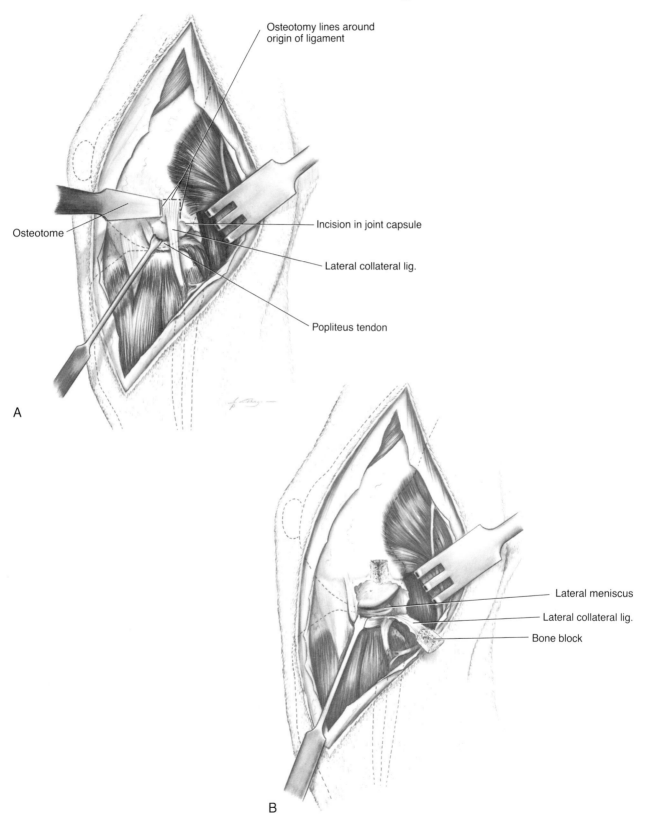

Osteotomy lines around origin of ligament

Osteotome

Incision in joint capsule

Lateral collateral lig.

Popliteus tendon

A

Lateral meniscus

Lateral collateral lig.

Bone block

B

Approach to the Medial Collateral Ligament and Caudomedial Part of the Stifle Joint

INDICATIONS

1. Removal of the caudal horn of the medial meniscus.
2. Repair of the medial collateral ligament.
3. Open reduction of fractures of caudal part of the medial femoral condyle.

ALTERNATIVE/COMBINATION APPROACHES

Plates 72, 73, 74, and 78

DESCRIPTION OF THE PROCEDURE

A. The skin incision extends from the distal fourth of the femur distally to the proximal fourth of the tibia, crossing the joint between the medial tibial condyle and tibial tuberosity. Subcutaneous tissues are incised on the same line and mobilized with the skin.

B. An incision is made in the deep fascia along the cranial border of the caudal part of the sartorius muscle.

Plate 77

Approach to the Medial Collateral Ligament and Caudomedial Part of the Stifle Joint

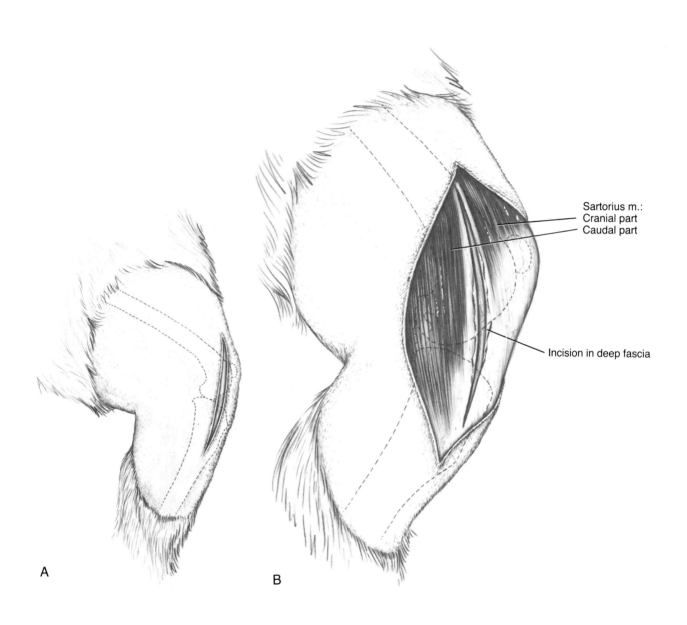

Sartorius m.:
Cranial part
Caudal part

Incision in deep fascia

A

B

Approach to the Medial Collateral Ligament and Caudomedial Part of the Stifle Joint *continued*

DESCRIPTION OF THE PROCEDURE *continued*

C. The caudal part of the sartorius muscle is retracted to expose the collateral ligaments. The joint capsule can be incised in a transverse direction on each side of the collateral ligament to expose the interior of the joint and the medial meniscus. Sharp dissection between the ligament and joint capsule is necessary in order to elevate it and protect it during the capsule incision.

CLOSURE

Interrupted absorbable sutures are placed in the joint capsule, and either continuous absorbable or interrupted nonabsorbable sutures are used to close the deep fascial incision. Subcutaneous tissues and skin are closed routinely.

COMMENTS

This approach is usually combined with the standard medial approach to the stifle (Plate 72) for total exposure of the stifle joint. The transverse joint capsule incision is an extension of the incision seen in Plate 72, Part C.

Plate 77

Approach to the Medial Collateral Ligament and Caudomedial Part of the Stifle Joint *continued*

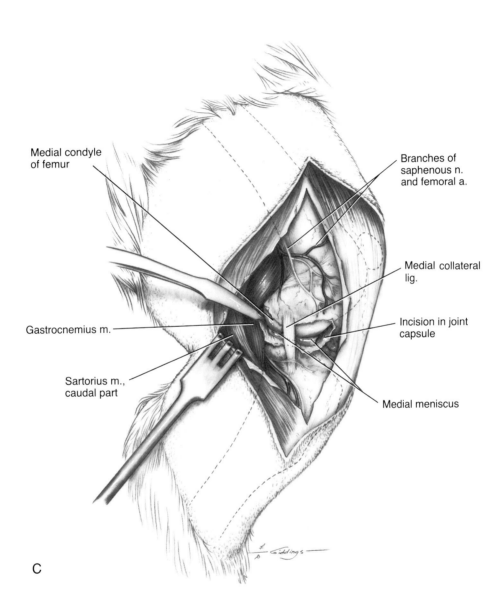

Medial condyle of femur

Branches of saphenous n. and femoral a.

Medial collateral lig.

Incision in joint capsule

Gastrocnemius m.

Sartorius m., caudal part

Medial meniscus

C

Approach to the Stifle Joint by Osteotomy of the Origin of the Medial Collateral Ligament
Based on a Procedure of Daly and Tarvin[8]

INDICATIONS

1. Reduction of fractures of the caudal part of the medial femoral condyle.
2. Exploration of the caudomedial part of the stifle joint.
3. Avulsion of the insertion of the caudal cruciate ligament.

ALTERNATIVE/COMBINATION APPROACHES

Plates 72, 73, 74, and 77

DESCRIPTION OF THE PROCEDURE

This procedure is a continuation of the Approach to the Medial Collateral Ligament and Caudomedial Part of the Stifle Joint (Plate 77).

A. After completely freeing the ligament from the joint capsule, an osteotome is used to outline a block of bone that contains the entire origin of the medial collateral ligament.

B. The block of bone is freed from the underlying condyle. Be sure to take an adequate amount of bone, because too small a block is difficult to fix securely in place. Note the wedge shape of the bone block; this will have some inherent stability when replaced. Abduction and external rotation of the tibia will expose the interior of the joint.

CLOSURE

The bone block origin of the ligament is reattached to the femur by means of a lag screw (Figure 24A). This can be simplified by predrilling before cutting the bone block. Interrupted sutures are placed in the joint capsule. The fascial incision is closed with either continuous absorbable or interrupted nonabsorbable sutures. Closure of the subcutaneous tissues and skin is routine.

Plate 78

Approach to the Stifle Joint by Osteotomy of the Origin of the Medial Collateral Ligament

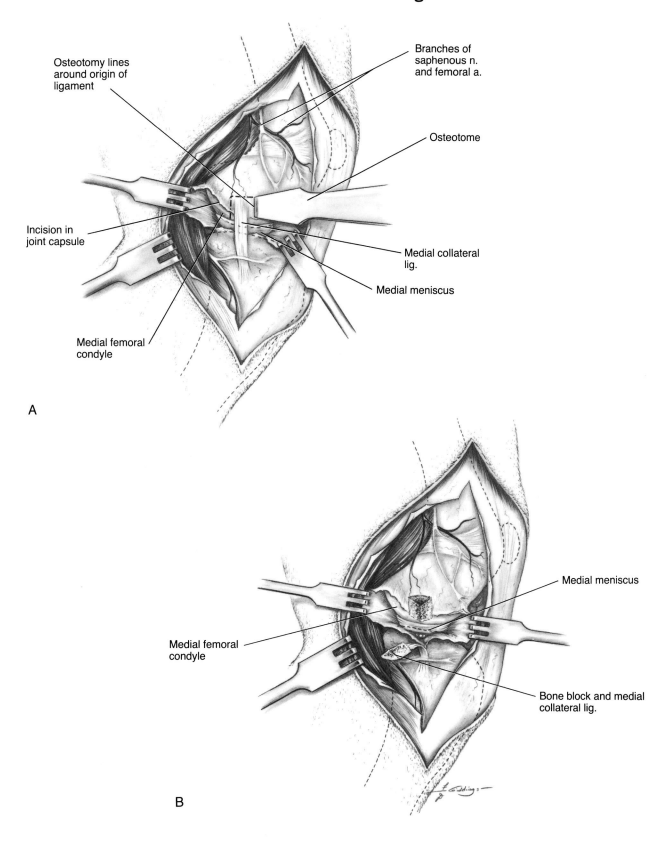

Osteotomy lines around origin of ligament

Branches of saphenous n. and femoral a.

Osteotome

Incision in joint capsule

Medial collateral lig.

Medial meniscus

Medial femoral condyle

A

Medial meniscus

Medial femoral condyle

Bone block and medial collateral lig.

B

Approach to the Shaft of the Tibia

Based on Procedures of Brinker[4] *and Wilson*[42]

INDICATION

Open reduction of fractures of the shaft of the tibia.

DESCRIPTION OF THE PROCEDURE

A. The skin incision can be varied to suit the situation. For maximal exposure of both the medial and lateral cortices and for bone plate application, the curved incision shown provides the best approach. A straight medial incision can be used for intramedullary pinning but would result in the plate being directly under the skin incision with only scanty subcuticular tissue to cover it if used in plating procedures. A curved, laterally based incision can be used if a plate is to be applied laterally.

The medially based incision shown here starts proximally over the medial tibial condyle and curves cranially to the midline of the tibia at midshaft. It then curves caudally to end near the medial malleolus. The subcutis is incised on the same line. Although not essential, an effort is made to preserve the saphenous vessels and nerve crossing the tibia.

B. The bone is exposed by incision of the crural fascia over the medial shaft of the bone. Elevating the fascia exposes the muscles.

C. The cranial tibial and medial digital flexor muscles can be retracted by incising fascia along their borders to free them from the bone.

Plate 79
Approach to the Shaft of the Tibia

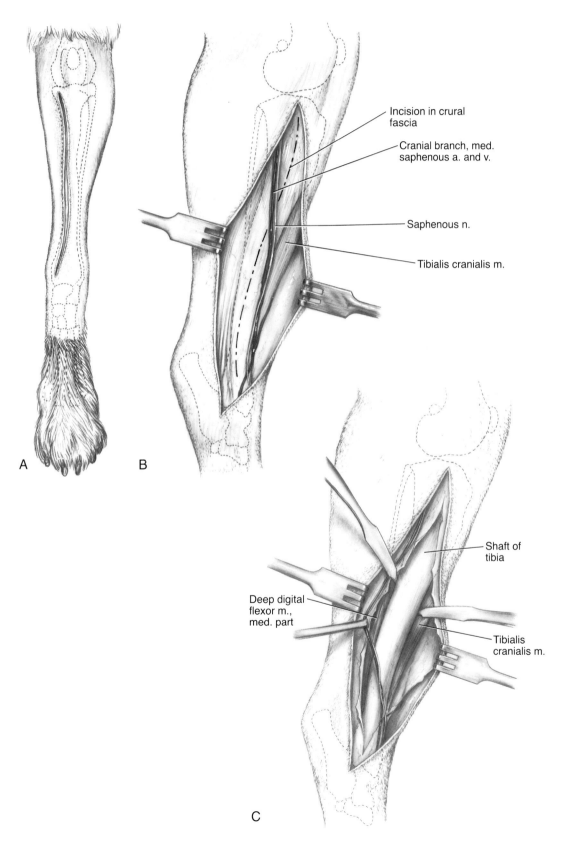

Incision in crural fascia

Cranial branch, med. saphenous a. and v.

Saphenous n.

Tibialis cranialis m.

Shaft of tibia

Deep digital flexor m., med. part

Tibialis cranialis m.

A

B

C

Approach to the Shaft of the Tibia *continued*

DESCRIPTION OF THE PROCEDURE *continued*

D. To expose the lateral cortex, the crural fascia is incised along the cranial border of the cranial tibial muscle, starting at the tibial tuberosity and extending distally to the tendinous portion of the muscle.

E. The cranial tibial and long digital extensor muscles are retracted caudolaterally to expose the tibial shaft. The cranial tibial artery courses between the tibia and fibula, and can be damaged by the Hohmann retractors' tips if they are placed over the artery.

Exposure of the distal lateral region of the tibia can be gained by incising fascia lateral to the tendons of the cranial tibial and long digital extensor muscles. Cranial retraction of these tendons provides visualization of the tibia.

CLOSURE

The deep crural fascia must be closed securely. Continuous absorbable or interrupted nonabsorbable sutures are used here and in the subcutaneous tissues. Skin and subcutis are closed routinely.

Plate 79

Approach to the Shaft of the Tibia *continued*

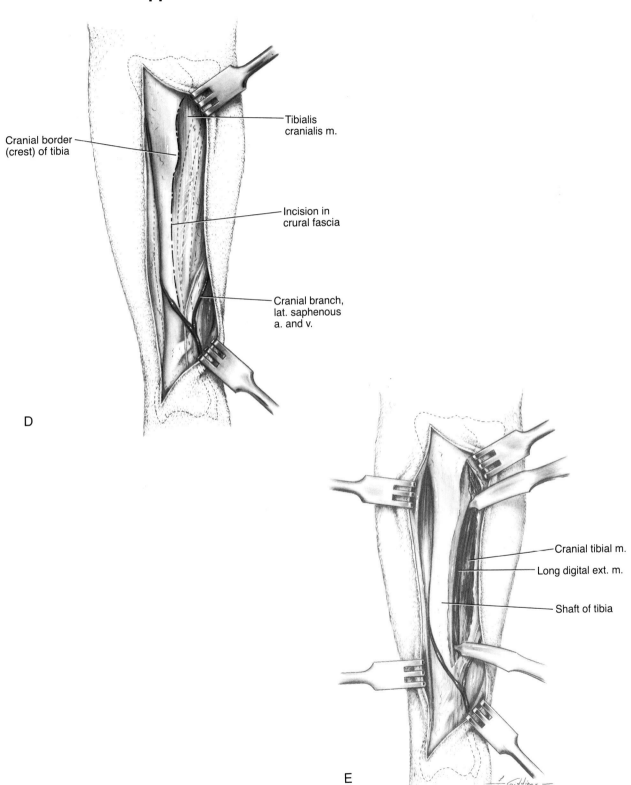

Cranial border (crest) of tibia

Tibialis cranialis m.

Incision in crural fascia

Cranial branch, lat. saphenous a. and v.

D

Cranial tibial m.

Long digital ext. m.

Shaft of tibia

E

Approach to the Lateral Malleolus and the Talocrural Joint

INDICATIONS

1. Open reduction of fractures of the lateral malleolus of the fibula.
2. Open reduction of supramalleolar fractures of the tibia.
3. Open reduction of luxations of the talocrural joint.
4. Repair of lateral collateral ligaments.
5. Osteochondroplasty for osteochondritis dissecans of the lateral trochlear ridge.

DESCRIPTION OF THE PROCEDURE

A. A curved skin incision is centered over the lateral surface of the talocrural joint. It commences proximally at the level of the lateral saphenous vein and continues distally to the level of the tarsometatarsal joint.

B. The subcutaneous and crural fascia is incised on the same line as the skin and is retracted with the skin. The extensor retinaculum overlying the lateral malleolus is incised parallel to the dorsal edge of the peroneus longus tendon, taking care to avoid cutting this small tendon. The tendon can now be retracted in any direction.

C. The lateral trochlear ridge of the talus is exposed by extending the joint and incising the joint capsule from the tibia distally, dorsal and parallel to the collateral ligament. This incision can be extended beyond what is shown here. The plantar aspect of the lateral talar ridge can be exposed by an incision in the joint capsule after retracting the tendons of the peroneus brevis and lateral digital extensor muscles and flexing the joint. A portion of the lateral extensor retinaculum must be elevated to make this incision and care must be taken to preserve as much as possible of the short, deep part of the lateral collateral ligament.

CLOSURE

The extensor retinaculum and joint capsule are closed with interrupted sutures. The crural and subcutaneous fascia is closed with a continuous pattern using absorbable sutures, followed by routine skin closure.

Plate 80

Approach to the Lateral Malleolus and Talocrural Joint

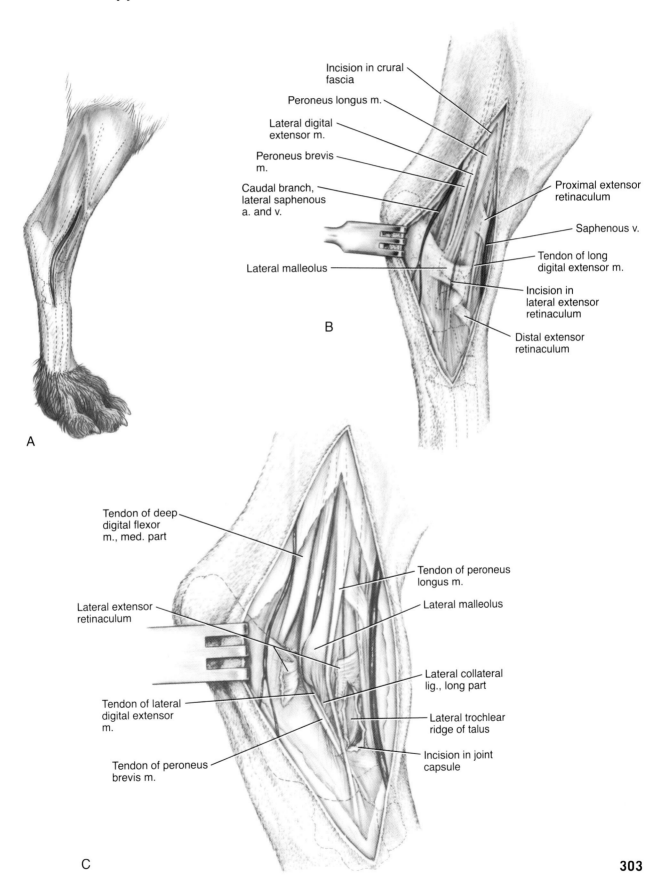

B

Incision in crural fascia

Peroneus longus m.

Lateral digital extensor m.

Peroneus brevis m.

Caudal branch, lateral saphenous a. and v.

Lateral malleolus

Proximal extensor retinaculum

Saphenous v.

Tendon of long digital extensor m.

Incision in lateral extensor retinaculum

Distal extensor retinaculum

A

C

Tendon of deep digital flexor m., med. part

Lateral extensor retinaculum

Tendon of lateral digital extensor m.

Tendon of peroneus brevis m.

Tendon of peroneus longus m.

Lateral malleolus

Lateral collateral lig., long part

Lateral trochlear ridge of talus

Incision in joint capsule

Approach to the Medial Malleolus and the Talocrural Joint

INDICATIONS

1. Open reduction of fractures of the medial malleolus of the fibula.
2. Open reduction of supramalleolar fractures of the tibia.
3. Open reduction of luxations of the talocrural joint.
4. Repair of medial collateral ligaments.
5. Osteochondroplasty for osteochondritis dissecans of the medial trochlear ridge.

DESCRIPTION OF THE PROCEDURE

A. A curved skin incision is centered over the medial surface of the talocrural joint. It commences proximally at the distal fourth of the tibia and continues distally to the level of the tarsometatarsal joint.

B. The subcutaneous and crural fascia is incised on the same line as the skin and is retracted with the skin. The medial ridge of the talus is exposed by a joint capsule incision that starts proximally on the tibia, continues parallel to the collateral ligament, and ends distally on the neck of the talus.

C. Retraction of the joint capsule and extension of the joint expose the dorsal aspect of the medial trochlear ridge of the talus. The plantar aspect of the ridge is accessed by a joint capsule incision plantar to the collateral ligament. The tendons of the tibialis caudalis and deep digital flexor muscles must be elevated and protected as this incision is made; this requires incising the overlying medial retinacular tissues parallel to the tendons. Varying degrees of flexion, extension, and rotation of the tarsus are required to visualize the talus.

CLOSURE

The extensor joint capsule incisions are closed with interrupted sutures. The crural and subcutaneous fascia are closed with a continuous pattern using absorbable sutures, followed by routine skin closure.

Plate 81

Approach to the Medial Malleolus and Talocrural Joint

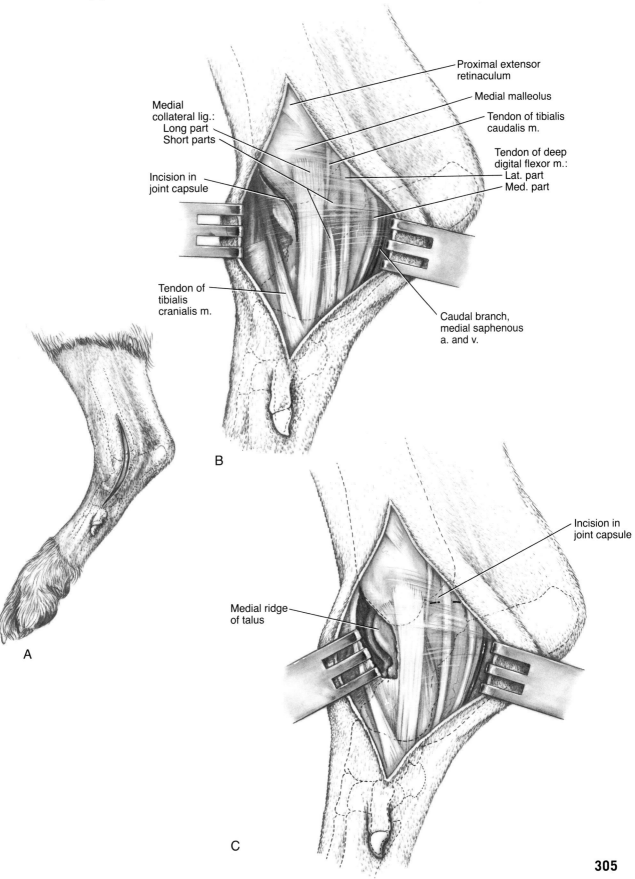

Proximal extensor retinaculum

Medial malleolus

Tendon of tibialis caudalis m.

Tendon of deep digital flexor m.:
Lat. part
Med. part

Medial collateral lig.:
Long part
Short parts

Incision in joint capsule

Tendon of tibialis cranialis m.

Caudal branch, medial saphenous a. and v.

A

B

Incision in joint capsule

Medial ridge of talus

C

305

Approach to the Tarsocrural Joint by Osteotomy of the Medial Malleolus

Based on a Procedure of Sinibaldi[34]

INDICATION

Open reduction of fractures of the trochlea of the talus.

ALTERNATIVE/COMBINATION APPROACH

Plate 81

DESCRIPTION OF THE PROCEDURE

This procedure is a continuation of the Approach to the Medial Malleolus and the Talocrural Joint (Plate 81).

A, B. The collateral ligament is isolated from joint capsule by incisions along the dorsal and plantar aspects of the ligament. These incisions should completely penetrate the joint capsule in order to allow sufficient visualization of the interior of the joint to judge the angle of the osteotomy, shown in Part B.

C. The medial malleolus is removed with an osteotome, placed as shown in Part B. The osteotomy angle should encompass enough of the malleolus to include most of the origin of the collateral ligament but must not be so deep as to intrude on the weight-bearing articular surface of the tibial cochlea. Care must also be taken to avoid cutting into the medial ridge of the talus. It may be necessary to incise part of the proximal extensor retinaculum to obtain the proper angle of the osteotome. Retraction of the malleolus and attached ligaments and pronation of the tarsus allow visualization of the entire surface of the trochlea of the talus.

CLOSURE

The malleolus is reattached with pins and tension band wire (Figure 23B) or a lag screw (Figure 24A). Interrupted sutures are used in the joint capsule, and a continuous pattern is used in the crural and subcutaneous fascia.

COMMENTS

Experience indicates that this approach is somewhat traumatic to the joint and should be reserved for trochlear fracture repair, where maximal exposure is necessary. Osteochondroplasty for osteochondritis dissecans of the talus is best done through the other approaches shown in Plates 80 and 81.

Plate 82

Approach to the Tarsocrural Joint by Osteotomy of the Medial Malleolus

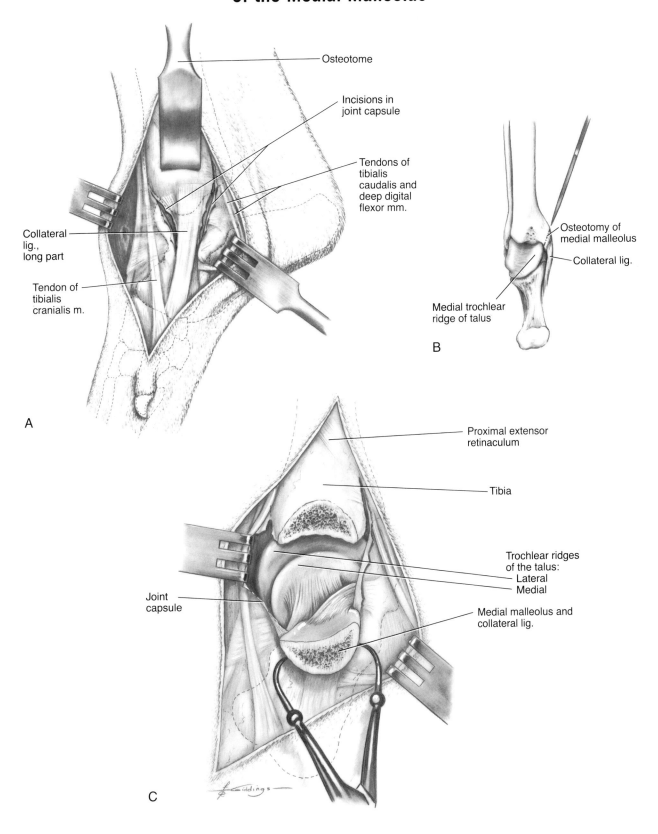

A

Osteotome

Incisions in joint capsule

Tendons of tibialis caudalis and deep digital flexor mm.

Collateral lig., long part

Tendon of tibialis cranialis m.

B

Osteotomy of medial malleolus

Collateral lig.

Medial trochlear ridge of talus

C

Proximal extensor retinaculum

Tibia

Trochlear ridges of the talus:
Lateral
Medial

Medial malleolus and collateral lig.

Joint capsule

Approach to the Calcaneus

INDICATIONS

1. Open reduction of fractures of the body and tuber calcanei of the calcaneus.
2. Avulsion of gastrocnemius tendon from tuber calcanei.

ALTERNATIVE/COMBINATION APPROACH

Plate 84

DESCRIPTION OF THE PROCEDURE

A. The skin incision begins on the lateral side of the common calcanean tendon just proximal to the tuber calcanei. As it curves distally, it remains lateral to the plantar midline of the calcaneus and ends at the level of the fourth tarsal bone.

B. The skin and thin subcutaneous fascia are reflected to expose the deep fascia. The lateral border of the tendon of the superficial digital flexor muscle is located by palpation or visualization through the fascia. An incision is made parallel to the lateral border of the tendon, through deep fascia and the lateral retinacular attachment of the tendon to the calcaneus, and is continued proximally to allow separation of the tendon from the gastrocnemius tendon.

C. Medial retraction of the tendon of the superficial digital flexor muscle completes the exposure.

CLOSURE

Interrupted, nonabsorbable sutures are used to approximate the deep fascial and retinacular incision. This part of the closure must be very secure to prevent the tendon from slipping medially over the calcaneus. Subcutis and skin are closed routinely.

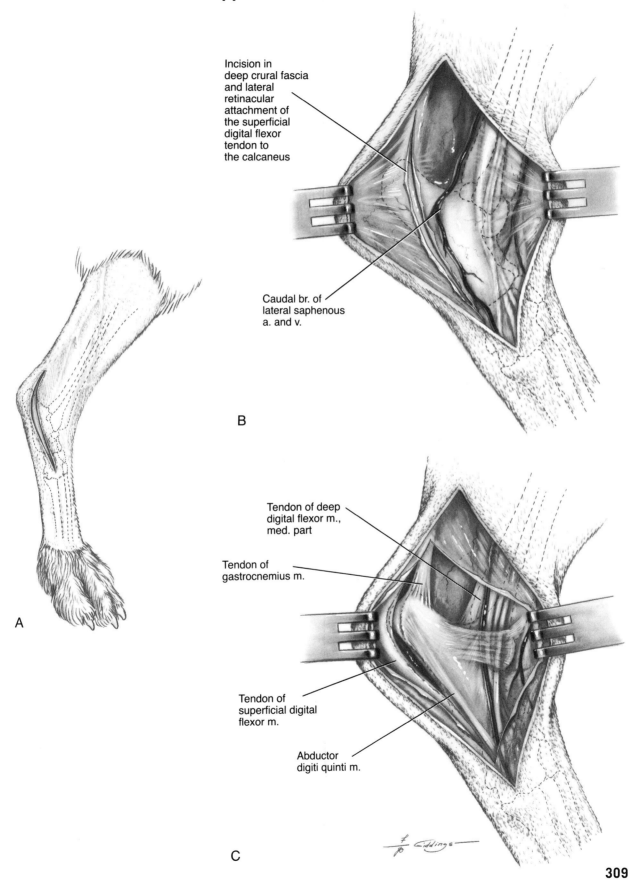

Plate 83
Approach to the Calcaneus

Incision in
deep crural fascia
and lateral
retinacular
attachment of
the superficial
digital flexor
tendon to
the calcaneus

Caudal br. of
lateral saphenous
a. and v.

B

Tendon of deep
digital flexor m.,
med. part

Tendon of
gastrocnemius m.

Tendon of
superficial digital
flexor m.

Abductor
digiti quinti m.

A

C

Approach to the Calcaneus and Plantar Aspects of the Tarsal Bones

INDICATION

Arthrodesis of the calcaneoquartile or tarsometatarsal joints.

DESCRIPTION OF THE PROCEDURE

This approach is based on the Approach to the Calcaneus (Plate 83).

A. Beginning on the lateral side of the common calcanean tendon, the skin incision curves ventrally along the calcaneus and then turns medially to cross the ventral midline at the level of the proximal metatarsal bones.

B. Elevation of the superficial digital flexor tendon is depicted in Plate 83, Parts B and C. The tendon is elevated distally to just beyond its bifurcation. A small branch of the plantar nerve will be found medial to the plantar midline in the fascia covering the deep digital flexor tendon. Incising this fascia lateral to the nerve will expose the deep digital flexor tendon.

C. The tendon of the deep digital flexor is elevated and retracted medially with the superficial tendon. The plantar ligament structure and tarsal bones come into view, but individual tarsal bones are difficult to discern visually. Probing with a needle will allow individual joint spaces to be located and incised.

CLOSURE

Interrupted, nonabsorbable sutures are used to approximate the deep fascial and retinacular incisions and bring both digital flexor tendons back to their normal positions.

Plate 84

Approach to the Calcaneus and Plantar Aspects
of the Tarsal Bones

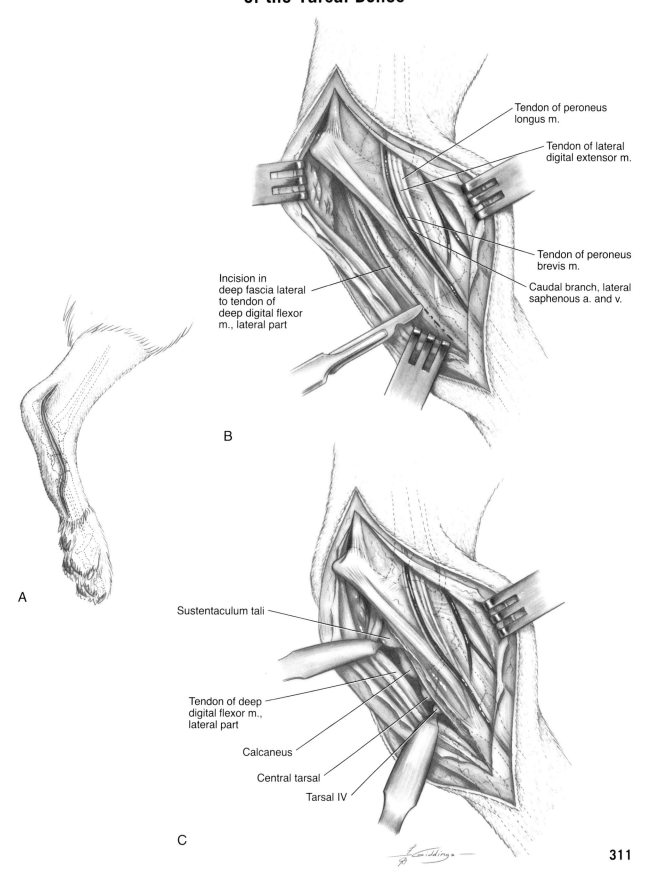

Tendon of peroneus
longus m.

Tendon of lateral
digital extensor m.

Tendon of peroneus
brevis m.

Caudal branch, lateral
saphenous a. and v.

Incision in
deep fascia lateral
to tendon of
deep digital flexor
m., lateral part

B

A

Sustentaculum tali

Tendon of deep
digital flexor m.,
lateral part

Calcaneus

Central tarsal

Tarsal IV

C

Approach to the Lateral Bones of the Tarsus

INDICATIONS

1. Open reduction of fractures or luxations of the base of the calcaneus or fourth tarsal bones.
2. Arthrodesis of the calcaneoquartile joint or lateral part of the tarsometatarsal joint.
3. Repair of injuries of the lateral ligaments of the calcaneoquartile joint or lateral part of the tarsometatarsal joint.

ALTERNATIVE/COMBINATION APPROACHES

Plates 80, 83, and 84

DESCRIPTION OF THE PROCEDURE

A. A lateral incision is made from midcalcaneus to the base of the fifth metatarsal bone.

B. The plantar metatarsal vessels can be seen in the deep fascia and positioned either superficial or plantar to the collateral ligaments of the tarsocrural joint. The deep fascia is incised dorsal to these vessels.

C. Retraction and elevation of the fascia reveal the underlying bones, tendons, and ligaments.

CLOSURE

Deep fascia is closed with interrupted sutures, followed by closure of the skin. There is usually insufficient subcutaneous tissue to close as a separate layer. A padded bandage should be used for several days to prevent serum accumulation in the subcutis.

Plate 85

Approach to the Lateral Bones of the Tarsus

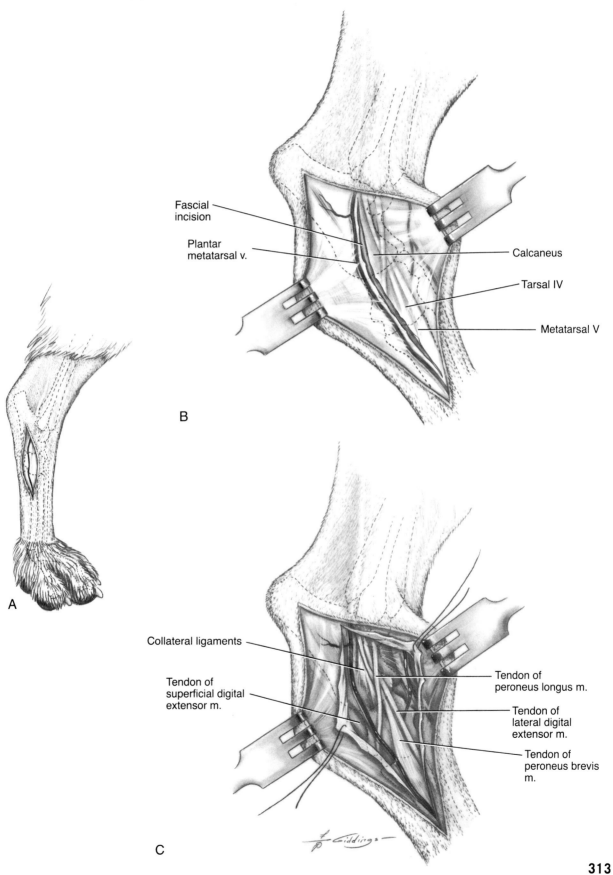

Fascial
incision

Plantar
metatarsal v.

Calcaneus

Tarsal IV

Metatarsal V

B

A

Collateral ligaments

Tendon of
superficial digital
extensor m.

Tendon of
peroneus longus m.

Tendon of
lateral digital
extensor m.

Tendon of
peroneus brevis
m.

C

Approach to the Medial Bones of the Tarsus

INDICATIONS

Open reduction of fractures or luxations of the neck and head of the talus, the central tarsal, or the second and third tarsal bones.

DESCRIPTION OF THE PROCEDURE

A. A vertical incision is made starting near the medial malleolus and extending to the base of metatarsal II. The length of the incision can be adjusted to fit the specific area of interest.

B. The subcutaneous fascia and skin are undermined and retracted. The deep fascia is incised between the tendon of the cranial tibial muscle and the branching metatarsal vessel from the saphenous vein. The metatarsal vein crossing the tendon is ligated.

C. The fascia lying on the surface of the tarsal bones is incised after retracting the tendon.

D. Elevation of the fascia reveals the tarsal bones and ligaments. A small Hohmann retractor can be placed under the fascia to expose the dorsal surface of the central tarsal. By keeping the elevation close to the bone, structures such as the dorsal pedal artery can be avoided.

CLOSURE

The deep fascia is joined by one row of interrupted sutures, followed by the skin. The subcutaneous tissues are usually too scant to require a separate layer. A padded bandage is used postoperatively for 5 to 7 days to prevent serum accumulation in the subcutis.

COMMENTS

Fractures of the central tarsal bone occur most commonly in track-raced greyhounds and usually in the right, or outside, foot.

Approach to the Proximal Sesamoid Bones

This procedure is identical to the approach to the proximal Sesamoid Bones illustrated in Plate 54 of Section V, The Forelimb.

Approach to the Phalanges and Interphalangeal Joints

This procedure is identical to the procedure illustrated in Plate 55 of Section V, The Forelimb.

Plate 86
Approach to the Medial Bones of the Tarsus

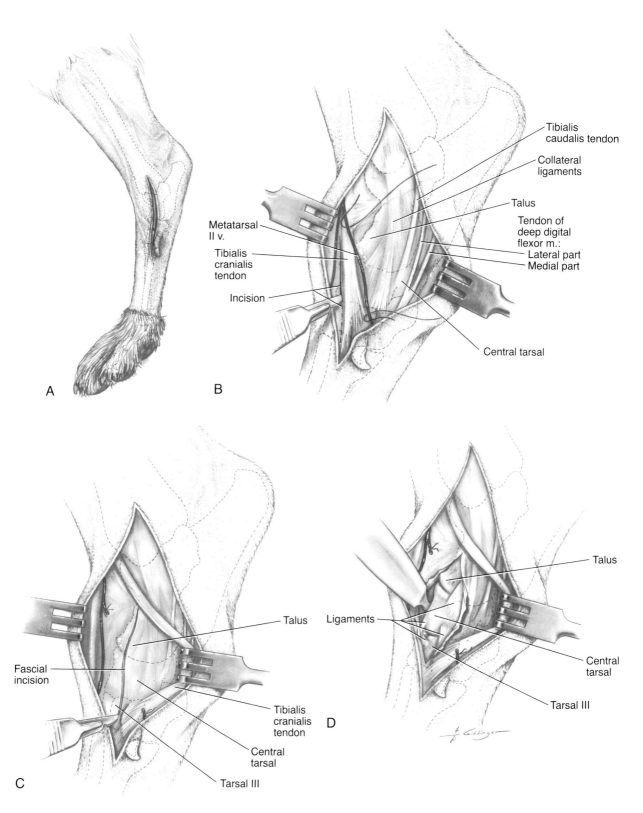

B

Tibialis caudalis tendon

Collateral ligaments

Talus

Tendon of deep digital flexor m.:
Lateral part
Medial part

Metatarsal II v.

Tibialis cranialis tendon

Incision

Central tarsal

A

C

Fascial incision

Talus

Tibialis cranialis tendon

Central tarsal

Tarsal III

D

Talus

Ligaments

Central tarsal

Tarsal III

Approaches to the Metatarsal Bones

INDICATION

Open reduction of fractures.

DESCRIPTION OF THE PROCEDURE

A. The anatomy shown here is considerably simplified compared to that in the live animal. Only important structures are shown; other elements such as small tendons and blood vessels have been omitted. In an average-sized dog, these vestigial structures are so small that their identification and preservation are not practical during surgery.

B, C, D. The incisional technique varies according to the bone or bones to be exposed. A single bone is approached by an incision directly over the bone, and two adjoining bones by an incision between them. If more than two bones need be exposed, two parallel longitudinal incisions (Part B) or a single curved incision (Part C) can be used. The curved incision commences at the proximal end of metatarsal II, runs laterally to the midshaft of metatarsal V, and then curves medially again to end over the distal end of metatarsal II. The crescent-shaped skin flap can be elevated and retracted to expose a large part of all four bones. An H-shaped incision (Part D) is useful on occasion.

Metatarsals II and V can be approached directly, without elevation of any important tendons or vessels. The deep fascia is incised and elevated to allow visualization of these bones. Exposure of metatarsal bones III and IV requires the undermining and retraction of the tendon of the long digital extensor tendons and the accompanying blood vessels.

CLOSURE

Deep fascia is closed to ensure that tendons and vessels are securely held in their proper positions.

COMMENTS

A deep layer of small metatarsal blood vessels is found on and between the bones. These vessels are too small to avoid in most animals, and the resulting hemorrhage must be controlled by tamponade. The use of an Esmarch bandage and a tourniquet is very helpful. Do not leave the tourniquet in place for more than 1½ hours, and apply a snug bandage for 72 hours postoperatively to control oozing hemorrhage at the operative site.

Plate 87

Approaches to the Metatarsal Bones

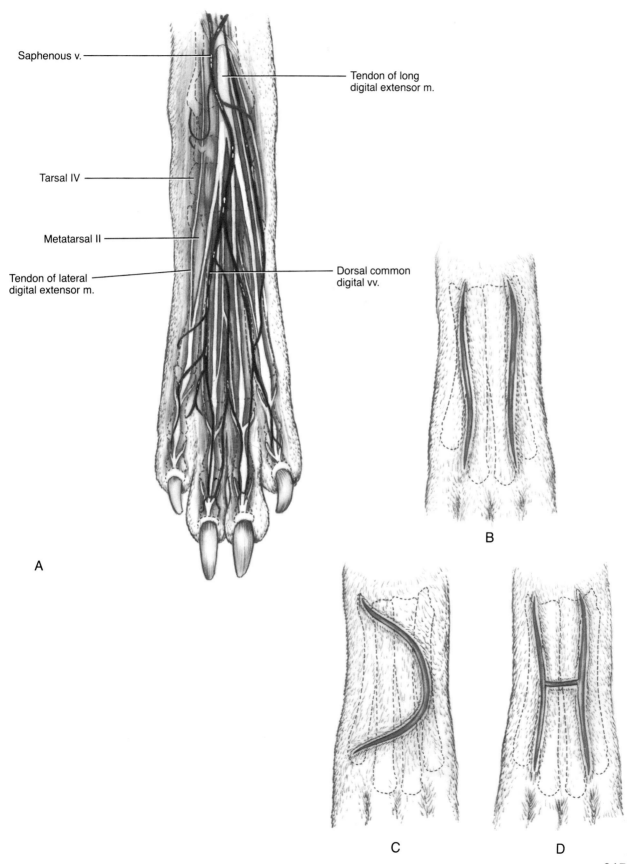

Saphenous v.

Tendon of long
digital extensor m.

Tarsal IV

Metatarsal II

Tendon of lateral
digital extensor m.

Dorsal common
digital vv.

A

B

C

D

References

1. Alexander JE: Open reduction and fixation of a shoulder luxation. *Sm Anim Clin* 2:379, 1962.
2. Alexander JE, Archibald J, Cawley AJ: Pelvic fractures and their reduction in small animals. *Mod Vet Pract* 43:41, 1962.
3. Archibald J, Brown NM, Nasti E, Medway W: Open reduction for correction of coxofemoral dislocation. *Vet Med* 48:273, 1953.
4. Brinker WO: Fractures. In Mayer K, Lacroix JV, Hoskins HP (eds): *Canine Surgery*, 4th ed. Santa Barbara: American Veterinary Publications, 1957, ch. 29.
5. Brown RE: A surgical approach to the coxofemoral joint of dogs. *North Am Vet* 34:420, 1953.
6. Brown SG, Rosen H: Craniolateral approach to the canine hip: A modified Watson-Jones approach. *J Am Vet Med Assoc* 159:1117, 1971.
7. Chalman JA, Slocum B: The caudolateral approach to the canine elbow joint. *J Am Anim Hosp Assoc* 19:637, 1983.
8. Daly WR, Tarvin GB: Medial condyle osteotomy as an approach to repair of medial condyle fractures in dogs. *Vet Surg* 10:119, 1981.
9. De Angelis M, Schwartz A: Surgical correction of a cranial dislocation of the scapulohumeral joint in a dog. *J Am Vet Med Assoc* 156:435, 1970.
10. Flo GL, Brinker WO: Lateral fenestration of thoracolumbar disc. *J Am Anim Hosp Assoc* 11:619, 1975.
11. Funkquist B: Decompression laminectomy for cervical disk protrusion in the dog. *Acta Vet Scand* 3:88, 1962.
12. Gahring DR: A modified caudal approach to the canine shoulder joint. *J Am Anim Hosp Assoc* 21:613, 1985.
13. Gorman HA: Hip joint prostheses. *Vet Scope* 7:3, #2, 1962.
14. Hoerlein BF, Few AB, Petty MF: Brain surgery in the dog—preliminary studies. *J Am Vet Med Assoc* 143:21, 1963.
15. Hohn RB: Surgical approaches to the canine hip. *Anim Hosp* 1:48, 1965.
16. Hohn RB: Osteochondritis dissecans of the humeral head. *J Am Vet Med Assoc* 163:69, 1973.
17. Hohn RB: Unpublished paper read at Fifth Annual course on Internal Fixation of Fractures, Ohio State University, Mar 27–30, 1974.
18. Hohn RB, Janes JM: Lateral approach to the canine ilium. *Anim Hosp* 2:111, 1966.
19. Hohn RB, Rosen H, Bohning RH, Brown SG: Surgical stabilization of recurrent shoulder luxation. *Vet Clin North Am* 1:537, 1971.
20. Hurov LI, Lumb WV, Hankes GH, Smith KW: Wedge grafting of the canine carpus. *J Am Vet Med Assoc* 148:260, 1966.
21. Lenehan TM, Nunamaker DM: Lateral approach to the canine elbow by proximal ulnar diaphyseal osteotomy. *J Am Vet Med Assoc* 180:523, 1982.
22. Montavon PM, Boudrieau RJ, Hohn RB: Ventrolateral approach for repair of sacroiliac fracture–dislocation in the dog and cat. *J Am Vet Med Assoc* 186:1198, 1985.
23. Montgomery RD, Milton JL, Mann FA: Medial approach to the humeral diaphysis. *J Am Anim Hosp Assoc* 24:433, 1988.
24. Mostosky UV, Cholvin NR, Brinker WO: Transolecranon approach to the elbow joint. *Vet Med* 54:560, 1959.
25. Nunamaker D: Personal communication, 1975.
26. Olsson SE: On disk protrusion in the dog. *Acta Orthop Scand* Suppl VIII, 1951.
27. Olsson SE: Lameness in the dog. *Sci Proc Am Anim Hosp Assoc* 1:366, 1975.
28. Paatsama S: Ligament injuries in the canine stifle joint: A clinical and experimental study. Thesis, Royal Veterinary College, Stockholm, 1952.
29. Parker A: Surgical approach to the cervicothoracic junction. *J Am Anim Hosp Assoc* 9:374, 1973.
30. Probst CW, Flo GL, McLoughlin MA, et al: A simple medial approach to the elbow for treatment of fragmented coronoid process and osteochondritis dissecans. *J Am Anim Hosp Assoc* 25:331, 1989.
31. Redding RW: Laminectomy in the dog. *Am J Vet Res* 12:123, 1951.
32. Rudy RL: Fractures of the maxilla and mandible. In Bojrab, J (ed): *Current Techniques in Small Animal Surgery*. Philadelphia: Lea & Febiger, 1975, p 369.
33. Seeman CW: A lateral approach for thoracolumbar disc fenestration. *Mod Vet Pract* 49:73, 1968.
34. Sinibaldi K: Unpublished paper read at 4th annual conference of the Vet Ortho Soc, Vail, CO, Feb 21–24, 1977.
35. Slocum B, Devine T: Pelvic osteotomy technique for axial rotation of the acetabular segment in dogs. *J Am Anim Hosp Assoc* 22:331, 1986.
36. Slocum B, Hohn RB: A surgical approach to the caudal aspect of the acetabulum and body of the ischium in the dog. *J Am Vet Med Assoc* 167:65, 1975.

37. Snavely DA, Hohn RB: A modified lateral surgical approach to the elbow of the dog. *J Am Vet Med Assoc* 169:826, 1977.

38. Sorjonen DC, Shires PK: Atlantoaxial instability: A ventral surgical technique for decompression, fixation, and fusion. *J Am Coll Vet Surg* 10:22, 1981.

39. Stoll SG: Unpublished paper read at 5th annual conference of the Vet Ortho Soc, Snowmass, CO, Feb 11–18, 1978.

40. Turner TM, Hohn RB: Craniolateral approach for repair of condylar fractures or joint exploration. *J Am Vet Med Assoc* 176:1264, 1980.

41. Wadsworth PL, Henry WB: Dorsal surgical approach to acetabular fractures in the dog. *J Am Med Assoc* 165:908, 1974.

42. Wilson JW: An anterior approach to the tibia. *J Am Anim Hosp Assoc* 10:67, 1974.

43. Yturraspe DJ, Lumb WV: Dorsolateral muscle separating approach for thoraco-lumbar intervertebral disk fenestration in the dog. *J Am Vet Med Assoc* 162:1037, 1973.

Index

Page numbers in *italics* refer to illustrations; those followed by the letter "t" refer to tables.

Abdominal oblique muscle, external, *25*
Abductor digiti quinti muscle, *29*
Abductor pollicis longus muscle, *26*
  tendon of, *27*
Absorbable suture materials, 22
Accessory carpal bone, approach to,
  210–212, *211, 213*
Acromion, *26*
  osteotomy of, 96
Alexander, Archibald, and Cawley
  procedure, for exposure of wing of
  ilium and dorsal sacrum, 222, *223*
Anatomy, 24
  of forelimb, *25, 26*
  of hindlimb, *27, 28, 29*
Anconeus muscle, *26*
Antibiotics, preoperative
  administration of, 3
Archibald, Brown, Nasti, and Medway
  procedure, for craniodorsal
  exposure of hip joint, 230–234, *231,*
  233, 235
Artery. See specific artery.
Aseptic technique, 3–14
Atlas. See also *Cervical vertebrae.*
  ventral approach to, 46–48, *47, 49*
  wings of, palpation of, 58
Autoclaving, 3
Axillary nerve, *26*
Axis. See also *Cervical vertebrae.*
  ventral approach to, 46–48, *47, 49*

Biceps brachii muscle, *25, 27*
Biceps femoris muscle, *28*
Bone. See specific bone.
Bone plating, 130
  palmar, 206
Brachial artery, *27*
Brachialis muscle, *25*
Braided suture materials, 22
Brain stem, caudal, exposure of, 42
Breed of animal, as factor in choosing
  approach, 2
Brinker procedure, for exposure of
  distal shaft and supracondylar
  region of humerus, 142–144, *143,*
  145

Brinker procedure *(Continued)*
  for exposure of distal shaft of humerus, 138–140, *139, 141*
  for exposure of femoral shaft, 270,
  271
  for exposure of tibial shaft, 298–300,
  299, 301
Brown procedure, for exposure of dorsal
  aspects of hip joint, 246, *247*
Brown and Rosen procedure, for
  craniodorsal exposure of hip joint,
  230–234, *231, 233, 235*
Bunnell-Mayer suture pattern, *20*

Calcaneus, approach to, 308, *309*
  plantar aspects of tarsus and, approach to, 310, *311*
Canine forequarter, subcutaneous
  musculature of, *25*
Canine hindquarter, deep musculature
  of, *29*
  subcutaneous musculature of, *28*
Canine thoracic limb, deep musculature
  of, *26, 27*
Carotid sheath, exposure of, 54, *55*
Carpus, dorsal approach to, 204, *205*
  palmarolateral approach to, 210–212,
  211, 213
  palmaromedial approach to, 206–208,
  207, 209
Cartilage fragments, in shoulder, 106,
  112
Caudal circumflex humeral artery, *26*
Caudal cutaneous sural nerve, *29*
Caudal vertebrae, dorsal approach to,
  88, *89*
Cephalic vein, *25, 27*
Cervical fascia, deep, exposure of, 54
Cervical spinal nerves, in canine
  thoracic limb, *27*
Cervical vertebrae, C1 and C2, dorsal
  approach to, 50–52, *51, 53*
  ventral approach to, 46–48, *47, 49*
  C2–C5, dorsal approach to, 60–62,
  61, 63
  C2–C7, ventral approach to, 54–58,
  55, 57, 59

Cervical vertebrae *(Continued)*
  C5–C7, dorsal approach to, 64–68,
  65, 67, 69
  palpation of, 58
Chalman and Slocum procedure, for
  exposure of elbow joint, 154–156,
  155, 157
Chlorhexidine, in skin disinfection, 4
Circumflex humeral arteries, *26*
Clavicular tendon, *25*
Cleidobrachialis muscle, *25*
Cleidocephalicus muscle, *25*
Clipping, as preparation for surgical
  procedures, 4
Closures, of different tissues, 23
  suture material used in, 22
Collateral ligament of stifle joint,
  lateral, approach to, 288, *289*
  medial, approach to, 292–294, *293,*
  295
Common digital extensor muscle, *26*
Common peroneal nerve, *29*
Coracobrachialis muscle, *27*
Cranial circumflex humeral artery, *26*
Cranial tibial muscle, *28, 29*
Cutaneous sural nerve, caudal, *29*

Daly and Tarvin procedure, for
  exposure of stifle joint, 296, *297*
De Angelis and Schwartz procedure, for
  exposure of shoulder joint, 118–
  120, *119, 121*
Deep digital flexor muscle, *27, 28, 29*
Deep gluteal muscle, *29*
Deep pectoral muscle, *25*
Deltoideus muscle, *25*
Dermal fat, closure of, 23, *24*
Digital extensor muscle, common, *26*
  lateral, *26*
  long, *28, 29*
Digital flexor muscle, deep, *27, 28, 29*
  superficial, *27, 28, 29*
Disks. See *Intervertebral disks.*
Draping, of animal, 5–14, *5–13*

Eighth cervical nerve, *27*

Elbow joint, approach to, by osteotomy of proximal ulnar diaphysis, 164–166, *165*, *167*
  caudal humeroulnar part of, approach to, 154–156, *155*, *157*
  exercises and weight bearing for, 166
  humeroradial part of, approach by osteotomy of lateral humeral epicondyle, 172–174, *173*, *175*
  humeroulnar part of, approach to, 158–162, *159*, *161*, *163*
  lateral humeroulnar part of, approach to, 150–152, *151*, *153*
  lateral parts of, approach to, 168–170, *169*, *171*
  medial aspect of, approach to, 176, *177*
Esophagus, exposure of, 54, *55*
Exercises and weight bearing, for elbow joint, 166
Extensor carpi radialis muscle, *26*, *27*
Extensor retinaculum, *29*
External abdominal oblique muscle, *25*
External jugular vein, *25*

Fascia, deep, closure of, 23
  incision of, *17*
  subcutaneous, closure of, 23, *24*
Fascia lata, *28*
Fat, dermal, closure of, 23, *24*
Femur, distal part of, approach through lateral incision, 272–274, *273*, *275*
  approach through osteotomy of tibial tuberosity, 286, *287*
  greater trochanter and subtrochanteric region of, approach to, 266–268, *267*, *269*
  shaft of, approach to, 270, *271*
First thoracic nerve, *27*
Flexor carpi radialis muscle, *27*
Flexor carpi ulnaris muscle, *26*
Flo and Brinker procedure, for exposure of thoracolumbar disks, 80–82, *81*, *83*
Forelimb. See *Thoracic limb.*
Forequarter, canine, deep musculature of, *26*, *27*
  subcutaneous musculature of, *25*
Fracture, type of, as factor in choosing approach, 3
Funkquist procedure, for exposure of vertebrae C1 and C2, 50–52, *51*, *53*
  for exposure of vertebrae C2–C5, 60–62, *61*, *63*

Gahring procedure, for exposure of shoulder joint, 108–112, *109*, *111*, *113*
Gastrocnemius muscle, *28*, *29*
Gemellus muscles, *29*
Gluteal muscle, deep, *29*
  middle, *28*
  superficial, *28*
Gorman procedure, for exposure of dorsal aspects of hip joint, 240–244, *241*, *243*, *245*
Gracilis muscle, *28*

Greater trochanter and subtrochanteric region of femur, approach to, 266–268, *267*, *269*

Head, surgical approaches to, 31–43
Hemilaminectomy, of thoracolumbar vertebrae, dorsal exposure for, 70–74, *71*, *73*, *75*
Hindlimb, 264–317
  anatomy of, *27*, *28*, *29*
Hindquarter, canine, deep musculature of, *29*
  subcutaneous musculature of, *28*
Hip bone, approach to, 252, *253*
Hip joint, 221–263
  craniodorsal and caudodorsal parts of, approach by osteotomy of greater trochanter, 240–244, *241*, *243*, *245*
    approach by tenotomy of gluteal muscles, 246, *247*
  craniodorsal aspect of, craniolateral approach to, 230–234, *231*, *233*, *235*
  dorsal aspect of, intergluteal approach to, 236–238, *237*, *239*
  ischium and, approach to, 248–250, *249*, *251*
  ventral aspect of, approach to, 254–256, *255*, *257*
Hoerlein, Few, and Petty procedure, for exposure of caudal surface of skull, 42, *43*
  for exposure of dorsolateral surface of skull, 40, *41*
Hohn procedure, for exposure of craniolateral shoulder joint, 98–100, *99*, *101*
  for exposure of elbow joint, 172–174, *173*, *175*
  for exposure of hip joint and ischium, 248–250, *249*, *251*
  for exposure of hip joint or ramus of pubis, 254–256, *255*, *257*
Hohn, Rosen, Bohning, and Brown procedure, for exposure of craniomedial shoulder joint, 114–116, *115*, *117*
Hohn and Janes procedure, for exposure of ilium, 224–226, *225*, *227*
Horizontal mattress suture pattern, *20*
Humeral arteries, circumflex, *26*
Humerus, approach for bone plating, 136
  condyle and epicondyle of, lateral approach to, 146–148, *147*, *149*
  condyle of, approach by osteotomy of medial epicondyle, 182–184, *183*, *185*
  distal shaft and supracondylar region of, medial approach to, 142–144, *143*, *145*
  distal shaft of, craniolateral approach to, 138–140, *139*, *141*
  full exposure of, 136
  lateral epicondyle of, osteotomy of, 172–174, *173*, *175*
  medial aspect of, intermuscular approach to, 178–180, *179*, *181*

Humerus *(Continued)*
  medial epicondyle of, approach to, 176, *177*
  proximal shaft of, approach to, 124–126, *125*, *127*
  shaft of, craniolateral approach to, 128–130, *129*, *131*
    medial approach to, 132–136, *133*, *135*, *137*
  supracondylar region of, approach to, 154–156, *155*, *157*
Hurov, Lumb, Hankes, and Smith procedure, for exposure of distal radius and carpus, 204, *205*

Iliocostalis muscle, *28*
Ilium, lateral approach to, 224–226, *225*, *227*
  wing of, approach to, 222, *223*
Infection, as factor in choosing approach, 3
Infraspinatus muscle, *26*
  tenotomy of, 98–100, *99*, *101*
Interior obturator muscle, tendon of, *29*
Internal jugular vein, exposure of, 54, *55*
Interphalangeal joints, of forelimb, approaches to, 218, *219*
  of hindlimb, approach to, 314
Intervertebral disks, C1–C2—C5–C6, ventral approach to, 54–58, *55*, *57*, *59*
  T10–T11—L5–L6, dorsolateral approach to, 76–78, *77*, *79*
  lateral approach to, 80–82, *81*, *83*
Intervertebral space, specific, location of, 58
Iodine, organic, in skin disinfection, 4
Ischium, approach to, 262, *263*
  hip joint and, approach to, 248–250, *249*, *251*
  tuberosity of, *29*

Joint. See specific joint.
Joint capsule, closure of, 23
Joint mice, in shoulder, 106
Jugular vein, external, *25*
  internal, exposure of, 54, *55*

Kessler (locking-loop) suture, *20*
Kirschner wire, for reattaching osteotomized bone, *20*

Lag screw, for reattaching osteotomized bone, *20*
Laminectomy, dorsal, 68
  of thoracolumbar vertebrae, dorsal exposure for, 70–74, *71*, *73*, *75*
Lateral collateral ligament of stifle joint, caudolateral stifle joint and, approach to, 288, *289*
Lateral digital extensor muscle, *26*
Lateral humeral epicondyle, osteotomy of, 172–174, *173*, *175*

Lateral malleolus, talocrural joint and, approach to, 302–304, *303, 305*
Lateral saphenous vein, *28*
Latissimus dorsi muscle, *25, 27*
Ligament(s). See also specific ligament. suturing of, *20,* 23
Locking-loop (Kessler) suture, *20*
Long digital extensor muscle, *28, 29*
Longissimus dorsi muscle, *28*
Lumbar vertebra(e), L7, dorsal approach to, 84–86, *85, 87, 89*
   L1–L3, dorsal approach to, 70–74, *71, 73, 75*

Mandible, caudal shaft and ramus of, approach to, 34, *35*
   ramus of, approach to, 36, *37*
   rostral shaft of, approach to, 32, *33*
Mattress suture pattern, horizontal, *20*
Medial collateral ligament of stifle joint, approach to, 292–294, *293, 295*
Medial coronoid process of ulna, approach to, by osteotomy of medial humeral epicondyle,182–184, *183, 185*
   intermuscular approach to, 178–180, *179, 181*
Medial humeral epicondyle, approach to, 176, *177*
Median nerve, *26, 27*
Metacarpal bones, approaches to, 214, *215*
Metacromion, in cat, 92, 96
Metatarsal bones, approaches to, 316, *317*
Middle gluteal muscle, *28*
Monofilament suture materials, 22
Montavon, Boudrieau, and Hohn procedure, for exposure of ventral aspect of sacrum, 228, *229*
Monteggia fracture, exposure for, 186
Montgomery, Milton, and Mann procedure, for exposure of shaft of humerus, 132–136, *133, 135, 137*
Mostosky, Cholvin, and Brinker procedure, for exposure of elbow joint, 158–162, *159, 161, 163*
Muscle(s). See also specific muscle.
   closure of, 23
   deep, of canine thoracic limb, *26, 27*
   elevation of, 16, 17, *18, 19*
   retraction of, 16, 22
   separation of, 16–17
   subcutaneous, of canine forequarter, *25*
   of canine hindquarter, *28*

Nerve. See specific nerve.
Nonabsorbable suture materials, 22

Obturator muscle, interior, tendon of, *29*
Occipital bone, open reduction of fractures of, 42, *43*
Olecranon. See *Elbow joint; Tuber olecrani.*

Omotransversarius muscle, *25*
Os coxae. See also *Ilium; Ischium; Pubis.*
   approach to, 252, *253*
Osteotomy, 19

Paatsama procedure, for exposure of distal femur and stifle joint, 272–274, *273, 275*
Palmar bone plating, 206
Palmar carpal region, superficial exposure of, 208
Palmarolateral carpal joints, approach to, 210–212, *211, 213*
Palpation, of vertebrae, 58
Parker procedure, for exposure of vertebrae C5–T3, 64–68, *65, 67*
Parotid salivary gland, *25*
Passive range of motion exercises, for elbow joint, 166
Pectineus muscle, *29*
Pectoral muscle, deep, *25*
   superficial, *25*
Pelvis, 221–263
   symphysis of, approach to, 258–260, *259, 261*
Peroneal nerve, common, *29*
Peroneus longus muscle, *28, 29*
Phalanges, of forelimb, approaches to, 218, *219*
   of hindlimb, approach to, 314
Pins, for reattaching osteotomized bone, *20*
Piriformis muscle, *29*
Popliteus muscle, *29*
Povidone iodine, for skin disinfection, 4
Probst et al. procedure, for exposure of medial elbow joint, 178–180, *179, 181*
Pronator teres muscle, *27*
Pubis, pelvic symphysis and, approach to, 258–260, *259, 261*
   ramus of, approach to, 254–256, *255, 257*
Pulley suture, *20*

Quadratus femoris muscle, *29*

Radial nerve, *26*
Radius, distal part of, dorsal approach to, 204, *205*
   palmaromedial approach to, 206–208, *207, 209*
   head and proximal metaphysis of, approach to, 192–194, *193, 195*
   head of, humeroradial part of elbow joint and, approach to, 172–174, *173, 175*
   lateral elbow joint and, approach to, 168–170, *169, 171*
   shaft of, lateral approach to, 200–202, *201, 203*
   medial approach to, 196–198, *197, 199,* 202
Range of motion exercises, for elbow joint, 166
Rectus femoris muscle, *29*

Redding procedure, for exposure of thoracolumbar vertebrae, 70–74, *71, 73, 75*
Retractors, types of, *16,* 22
Rhomboid muscle, attachment of, *27*
Rudy procedure, for exposure of rostral shaft of mandible, 32, *33*

Sacroiliac joint, direct visualization of, 228
Sacrotuberous ligament, *29*
Sacrum, approach to dorsal aspect of, 222, *223*
   approach to ventral aspect of, 228, *229*
   vertebra L7 and, dorsal approach to, 84–86, *85, 87, 89*
Salivary gland, parotid, *25*
Saphenous vein, lateral, *28*
Sartorius muscle, *28*
Scapula, body, spine, and acromion process of, approach to, 92, *93*
   neck and glenoid cavity of, approach to, 120
Sciatic nerve, *29*
Seeman procedure, for exposure of thoracolumbar disks, 80–82, *81, 83*
Semimembranosus muscle, *28, 29*
Semitendinosus muscle, *28, 29*
Serratus ventralis muscle, attachment of, *27*
Sesamoid bones, of forelimb, approach to, 216, *217*
   of hindlimb, approach to, 314
Seventh cervical nerve, in canine thoracic limb, *27*
Shoulder joint, caudal region of, approach to, 108–112, *109, 111, 113*
   caudolateral region of, approach to, 102–106, *103, 105, 107*
   cranial region of, approach to, 118–120, *119, 121*
   craniolateral region of, approach to, 94–96, *95, 97,* 98–100, *99, 101*
   craniomedial region of, approach to, 114–116, *115, 117*
   exposure of, for removal of cartilage fragments, 106, 112
Sinibaldi, procedure of, for exposure of tarsocrural joint, 306, *307*
Sixth cervical nerve, in canine thoracic limb, *27*
Skin, closure of, 23
   disinfection of, 4
   incision and retraction of, 15
   preparation of, for surgical procedures, 3–5
Skull, caudal surface of, approach to, 42, *43*
   dorsolateral surface of, approach to, 40, *41*
Slocum and Devine procedure, for exposure of ventral aspect of hip joint or pubic ramus, 254–256, *255, 257*
Slocum and Hohn procedure, for exposure of hip joint and ischium, 248–250, *249, 251*

Snavely and Hohn procedure, for exposure of elbow joint, 150–152, *151, 153*
Soft-tissue damage, as factor in choosing approach, 3
Sorjonen and Shires procedure, for exposure of vertebrae C1 and C2, 46–48, *47, 49*
Spinal column. See also *Vertebra(e).*
    surgical approaches to, 45–67
Spinal cord, cranial, exposure of, 42
Spinal nerves, in canine thoracic limb, *27*
Sterilization, of surgical supplies, 3
Sternocephalicus muscle, *25*
Sternohyoideus muscle, *25*
Stifle joint, approach through osteotomy of lateral collateral ligament, 290, *291*
    approach through osteotomy of medial collateral ligament, 296, *297*
    bilateral approach to, 274, 282–284, *283, 285*
    caudolateral part of, approach to, 288, *289*
    caudomedial part of, approach to, 292–294, *293, 295*
    distal femur and, approach through lateral incision, 272–274, *273, 275*
        approach through osteotomy of tibial tuberosity, 286, *287*
    lateral approach to, 276, *277*
    lateral collateral ligament of, approach to, 288, *289*
    medial approach to, 278–280, *279, 281*
    medial collateral ligament of, approach to, 292–294, *293, 295*
    total exposure of, 294
Stirrup, for suspension of limb, 4, *4*
Stockinette, for surgical procedures, 4, 6, *6, 7, 8, 9, 10, 11, 12, 13*
Stoll procedure, for exposure of medial elbow joint, 182–184, *183, 185*
Subcutaneous fascia, closure of, 23, *24*
Subcutaneous musculature, of canine forequarter, *25*
    of canine hindquarter, *28*
Subcutaneous tissue, incision and retraction of, 15–16
    suturing of, *24*
Subscapular artery, *26*
Subscapularis muscle, *27*
Superficial digital flexor muscle, *27, 28, 29*
Superficial gluteal muscle, *28*
Superficial pectoral muscle, *25*
Supraspinatus muscle, *26, 27*
Sural nerve, caudal cutaneous, *29*

Surgery, principles of, 14–24
Suspension of limb, stirrup for, 4, *4*
Suture materials, 22
Suturing, of different tissues, 20, 23
    patterns for, *20*

Talocrural joint, lateral malleolus and, approach to, 302–304, *303, 305*
Tarsocrural joint, approach by osteotomy of medial malleolus, 306, *307*
Tarsus, lateral bones of, approach to, 312, *313*
    medial bones of, approach to, 314, *315*
    plantar aspects of, approach to, 310, *311*
Temporomandibular joint, 36
Tendon(s). See also specific tendon.
    closure of, 23
    suturing of, 19, *20*
Tenotomy, 19
Tension band wire, for reattaching osteotomized bone, *20*
Tensor fasciae antebrachii muscle, *27*
Tensor fasciae latae muscle, *28, 29*
Teres major muscle, *27*
Teres minor muscle, *26*
Thoracic limb, approaches to, 122–219
    canine, deep musculature of, *26, 27*
    subcutaneous musculature of, *25*
Thoracic spinal nerve, *27*
Thoracic vertebrae, T1–T3, dorsal approach to, 64–68, *65, 67, 69*
    T12 and T13, dorsal approach to, 70–74, *71, 73, 75*
Thoracolumbar intervertebral disks (T10–T11—L5–L6), dorsolateral approach to, 76–78, *77, 79*
    lateral approach to, 80–82, *81, 83*
Thoracolumbar vertebrae (T12–L3), dorsal approach to, 70–74, *71, 73, 75*
Tibia, shaft of, approach to, 298–300, *299, 301*
Tibial muscle, cranial, *28, 29*
Tibial nerve, *29*
Tissue damage, as factor in choosing approach, 3
Trachea, exposure of, 54, *55*
Trapezius muscle, *25*
Triceps brachii muscle, *25, 27*
Trochanter, greater, *29*
    approach to, 266–268, *267, 269*
Trochlear notch of ulna, approach to, 186, *187*
Tuber olecrani, approach to, 188, *189*
    osteotomy of, 158–162, *159, 161, 163*

Tuberosity of ischium, *29*
Turner and Hohn procedure, for exposure of elbow joint, 146–148, *147, 149*

Ulna, distal shaft and styloid process of, approach to, 190, *191*
    medial coronoid process of, approach to, 182–184, *183, 185*
        intermuscular approach to, 178–180, *179, 181*
    proximal diaphysis of, osteotomy of, 164–166, *165, 167*
    proximal shaft and trochlear notch of, approach to, 186, *187*
Ulnar nerve, *26, 27*
Ulnaris lateralis muscle, *26*

Vastus lateralis muscle, *29*
Vastus medialis muscle, *28, 29*
Vein. See specific vein.
Vertebra(e). See also *Atlas; Axis.*
    C1 and C2, dorsal approach to, 50–52, *51, 53*
        ventral approach to, 46–48, *47, 49*
    C2–C5, dorsal approach to, 60–62, *61, 63*
    C2–C7, ventral approach to, 54–58, *55, 57, 59*
    C5–T3, dorsal approach to, 64–68, *65, 67, 69*
    caudal, approach to, 88, *89*
    L7, dorsal approach to, 84–86, *85, 87, 89*
    numbering of, 58, 82
    T12–L3, dorsal approach to, 70–74, *71, 73, 75*
Vertebral column, surgical approaches to, 45–67

Wadsworth and Henry procedure, for exposure of dorsal aspect of hip joint, 236–238, *237, 239*
Weight bearing and exercises, for elbow joint, 166
Wilson procedure, for exposure of tibial shaft, 298–300, *299, 301*
Wires, for reattaching osteotomized bone, *20*

Yturraspe and Lumb procedure, for exposure of thoracolumbar disks, 76–78, *77, 79*